HEALTH AND HUMAN DEVELOPMENT

PSYCHOSOCIAL NEEDS

SUCCESS IN LIFE AND CAREER PLANNING

HEALTH AND HUMAN DEVELOPMENT
JOAV MERRICK - SERIES EDITOR
NATIONAL INSTITUTE OF CHILD HEALTH AND HUMAN DEVELOPMENT, MINISTRY OF SOCIAL AFFAIRS, JERUSALEM

Psychosocial Needs: Success in Life and Career Planning
Daniel TL Shek, Janet TY Leung, Tak-yan Lee, and Joav Merrick (Editors)
2017. ISBN: 978-1-53611-951-0 (Hardcover)
2017. ISBN: 978-1-53611-971-8 (eBook)

Palliative Care: Psychosocial and Ethical Considerations
Blair Henry, Arnav Agarwal, Edward Chow, and Joav Merrick (Editors)
2017. ISBN: 978-1-53610-607-7 (Hardcover)
2017. ISBN: 978-1-53610-611-4 (eBook)

Cannabis: Medical Aspects
Blair Henry, Arnav Agarwal, Edward Chow, Hatim A Omar, and Joav Merrick (Editors)
2017. ISBN: 978-1-53610-510-0 (Hardcover)
2017. ISBN: 978-1-53610-522-3 (eBook)

Public Health Yearbook 2016
Joav Merrick (Editor)
2017. ISBN: 978-1-53610-947-4 (Hardcover)
2017. ISBN: 978-1-53610-956-6 (eBook)

Alternative Medicine Research Yearbook 2016
Joav Merrick (Editor)
2017. ISBN: 978-1-53610-972-6 (Hardcover)
2017. ISBN: 978-1-53611-000-5 (eBook)

Oncology: The Promising Future of Biomarkers
Anthony Furfari,
George S Charames,
Rachel McDonald,
Leigha Rowbottom,
Azar Azad, Stephanie Chan,
Bo Angela Wan, Ronald Chow,
Carlo DeAngelis, Pearl Zaki,
Edward Chow and Joav Merrick
(Editors)
2017. ISBN: 978-1-53610-608-4
(Hardcover)
2017. ISBN: 978-1-53610-610-7
(eBook)

Pain Management Yearbook 2016
Joav Merrick (Editor)
2017. ISBN: 978-1-53610-949-8
(Hardcover)
2017. ISBN: 978-1-53610-959-7
(eBook)

Medical Cannabis: Clinical Practice
Shannon O'Hearn, Alexia Blake,
Bo Angela Wan, Stephanie Chan,
Edward Chow and Joav Merrick
(Editors)
2017. ISBN: 978-1-53611-907-7
(Softcover)
2017. ISBN: 978-1-53611-927-5
(eBook)

Cancer: Treatment, Decision Making and Quality of Life
Breanne Lechner, Ronald Chow,
Natalie Pulenzas, Marko Popovic,
Na Zhang, Xiaojing Zhang,
Edward Chow, and Joav Merrick
(Editors)
2016. ISBN: 978-1-63483-863-4
(Hardcover)
2015. ISBN: 978-1-63483-882-5
(eBook)

Cancer: Bone Metastases, CNS Metastases and Pathological Fractures
Breanne Lechner, Ronald Chow,
Natalie Pulenzas, Marko Popovic,
Na Zhang, Xiaojing Zhang,
Edward Chow, and Joav Merrick
(Editors)
2016. ISBN: 978-1-63483-949-5
(Hardcover)
2015. ISBN: 978-1-63483-960-0
(eBook)

Cancer: Spinal Cord, Lung, Breast, Cervical, Prostate, Head and Neck Cancer
Breanne Lechner, Ronald Chow, Natalie Pulenzas, Marko Popovic, Na Zhang, Xiaojing Zhang, Edward Chow and Joav Merrick (Editors)
2016. ISBN: 978-1-63483-904-4 (Hardcover)
2015. ISBN: 978-1-63483-911-2 (eBook)

Cancer: Survival, Quality of Life and Ethical Implications
Breanne Lechner, Ronald Chow, Natalie Pulenzas, Marko Popovic, Na Zhang, Xiaojing Zhang, Edward Chow and Joav Merrick (Editors)
2016. ISBN: 978-1-63483-905-1 (Hardcover)
2015. ISBN: 978-1-63483-912-9 (eBook)

Cancer: Pain and Symptom Management
Breanne Lechner, Ronald Chow, Natalie Pulenzas, Marko Popovic, Na Zhang, Xiaojing Zhang, Edward Chow, and Joav Merrick (Editors)
2016. ISBN: 978-1-63483-905-1 (Hardcover)
2015. ISBN: 978-1-63483-881-8 (eBook)

Alternative Medicine Research Yearbook 2015
Joav Merrick (Editor)
2016. ISBN: 978-1-63484-511-3 (Hardcover)
2016. ISBN: 978-1-63484-542-7 (eBook)

Public Health Yearbook 2015
Joav Merrick (Editor)
2016. ISBN: 978-1-63484-511-3 (Hardcover)
2016. ISBN: 978-1-63484-546-5 (eBook)

Quality, Mobility and Globalization in the Higher Education System: A Comparative Look at the Challenges of Academic Teaching
Nitza Davidovitch, Zehavit Gross, Yuri Ribakov, and Anna Slobodianiuk (Editors)
2016. ISBN: 978-1-63484-986-9 (Hardcover)
2016. ISBN: 978-1-63485-012-4 (eBook)

Alternative Medicine Research Yearbook 2014
Joav Merrick (Editor)
2015. ISBN: 978-1-63482-161-2 (Hardcover)
2015. ISBN: 978-1-63482-205-3 (eBook)

Pain Management Yearbook 2014
Joav Merrick (Editor)
2015. ISBN: 978-1-63482-164-3
(Hardcover)
2015. ISBN: 978-1-63482-208-4
(eBook)

Public Health Yearbook 2014
Joav Merrick (Editor)
2015. ISBN: 978-1-63482-165-0
(Hardcover)
2015. ISBN: 978-1-63482-209-1
(eBook)

Forensic Psychiatry:
A Public Health Perspective
Leo Sher and Joav Merrick (Editors)
2015. ISBN: 978-1-63483-339-4
(Hardcover)
2015. ISBN: 978-1-63483-346-2
(eBook)

Leadership and Service Learning Education: Holistic Development for Chinese University Students
Daniel TL Shek, Florence KY Wu and Joav Merrick (Editors)
2015. ISBN: 978-1-63483-340-0
(Hardcover)
2015. ISBN: 978-1-63483-347-9
(eBook)

Mental and Holistic Health:
Some International Perspectives
Joseph L Calles Jr,
Donald E Greydanus,
and Joav Merrick (Editors)
2015. ISBN: 978-1-63483-589-3
(Hardcover)
2015. ISBN: 978-1-63483-608-1
(eBook)

India: Health and Human Development Aspects
Joav Merrick (Editor)
2014. ISBN: 978-1-62948-784-7
(Hardcover)
2014. ISBN: 978-1-62948-794-6
(eBook)

Alternative Medicine Research Yearbook 2013
Joav Merrick (Editor)
2014. ISBN: 978-1-63321-094-3
(Hardcover)
2014. ISBN: 978-1-63321-144-5
(eBook)

Health Consequences of Human Central Obesity
Kaushik Bose and Raja Chakraborty (Editors)
2014. ISBN: 978-1-63321-152-0
(Hardcover)
2014. ISBN: 978-1-63321-181-0
(eBook)

Public Health Yearbook 2013
Joav Merrick (Editor)
2014. ISBN: 978-1-63321-095-0
(Hardcover)
2014. ISBN: 978-1-63321-097-4
(eBook)

Public Health: Improving Health via Inter-Professional Collaborations
Rosemary M Caron and Joav Merrick (Editors)
2014. ISBN: 978-1-63321-569-6
(Hardcover)
2014. ISBN: 978-1-63321-594-8
(eBook)

Health and Happiness from Meaningful Work: Research in Quality of Working Life
Søren Ventegodt and Joav Merrick (Editors)
2013. ISBN: 978-1-60692-820-2
(Hardcover)
2009. ISBN: 978-1-61324-981-9
(eBook)

Adolescence and Sports
Dilip R Patel, Donald E Greydanus, Hatim Omar and Joav Merrick (Editors)
2013. ISBN: 978-1-60876-702-1
(Hardcover)
2010. ISBN: 978-1-61761-483-5
(eBook)

Textbook on Evidence-Based Holistic Mind-Body Medicine: Holistic Practice of Traditional Hippocratic Medicine
Søren Ventegodt and Joav Merrick
2013. ISBN: 978-1-62257-105-5
(Hardcover)
2012. ISBN: 978-1-62257-174-1
(eBook)

Textbook on Evidence-Based Holistic Mind-Body Medicine: Healing the Mind in Traditional Hippocratic Medicine
Søren Ventegodt and Joav Merrick
2013. ISBN: 978-1-62257-112-3
(Hardcover)
2012. ISBN: 978-1-62257-175-8
(eBook)

Textbook on Evidence-Based Holistic Mind-Body Medicine: Sexology and Traditional Hippocratic Medicine
Søren Ventegodt and Joav Merrick
2013. ISBN: 978-1-62257-130-7
(Hardcover)
2012. ISBN: 978-1-62257-176-5
(eBook)

Conceptualizing Behavior in
Health and Social Research:
A Practical Guide to Data
Analysis
*Said Shahtahmasebi
and Damon Berridge*
2013. ISBN: 978-1-60876-383-2

Pediatric and Adolescent
Sexuality and Gynecology:
Principles for the Primary
Care Clinician
*Hatim A Omar,
Donald E Greydanus,
Artemis K Tsitsika, Dilip R Patel
and Joav Merrick (Editors)*
2013. ISBN: 978-1-60876-735-9
(Softcover)

Human Development: Biology
from a Holistic Point of View
*Søren Ventegodt,
Tyge Dahl Hermansen
and Joav Merrick*
2013. ISBN: 978-1-61470-441-6
(Hardcover)
2011. ISBN: 978-1-61470-541-3
(eBook)

Building Community Capacity:
Case Examples from Around
the World
*Rosemary M Caron and Joav Merrick
(Editors)*
2013. ISBN: 978-1-62417-175-8
(Hardcover)
2013. ISBN: 978-1-62417-176-5
(eBook)

Managed Care in a Public Setting
Richard Evan Steele
2013. ISBN: 978-1-62417-970-9
(Softcover)
2013. ISBN: 978-1-62417-863-4
(eBook)

Bullying:
A Public Health Concern
*Jorge C Srabstein and Joav Merrick
(Editors)*
2013. ISBN: 978-1-62618-564-7
(Hardcover)
2013. ISBN: 978-1-62618-588-3
(eBook)

Bedouin Health: Perspectives
from Israel
*Joav Merrick, Alean Al-Krenami
and Salman Elbedour (Editors)*
2013. ISBN: 978-1-62948-271-2
(Hardcover)
2013: ISBN: 978-1-62948-274-3
(eBook)

Health Promotion: Community Singing as a Vehicle to Promote Health
Jing Sun, Nicholas Buys and Joav Merrick (Editors)
2013. ISBN: 978-1-62618-908-9 (Hardcover)
2013: ISBN: 978-1-62808-006-3 (eBook)

Public Health Yearbook 2012
Joav Merrick (Editor)
2013. ISBN: 978-1-62808-078-0 (Hardcover)
2013: ISBN: 978-1-62808-079-7 (eBook)

Alternative Medicine Research Yearbook 2012
Joav Merrick (Editor)
2013. ISBN: 978-1-62808-080-3 (Hardcover)
2013: ISBN: 978-1-62808-079-7 (eBook)

Advanced Cancer: Managing Symptoms and Quality of Life
Natalie Pulenzas, Breanne Lechner, Nemica Thavarajah, Edward Chow, and Joav Merrick (Editors)
2013. ISBN: 978-1-62808-239-5 (Hardcover)
2013: ISBN: 978-1-62808-267-8 (eBook)

Treatment and Recovery of Eating Disorders
Daniel Stein and Yael Latzer (Editors)
2013. ISBN: 978-1-62808-248-7 (Softcover)

Health Promotion: Strengthening Positive Health and Preventing Disease
Jing Sun, Nicholas Buys and Joav Merrick (Editors)
2013. ISBN: 978-1-62257-870-2 (Hardcover)
2013: ISBN: 978-1-62808-621-8 (eBook)

Pain Management Yearbook 2011
Joav Merrick (Editor)
2013. ISBN: 978-1-62808-970-7 (Hardcover)
2013: ISBN: 978-1-62808-971-4 (eBook)

Pain Management Yearbook 2012
Joav Merrick (Editor)
2013. ISBN: 978-1-62808-973-8 (Hardcover)
2013: ISBN: 978-1-62808-974-5 (eBook)

Suicide from a Public Health Perspective
Said Shahtahmasebi and Joav Merrick
2013. ISBN: 978-1-62948-536-2 (Hardcover)
2014: ISBN: 978-1-62948-537-9 (eBook)

Food, Nutrition and Eating Behavior
Joav Merrick and Sigal Israeli (Editors)
2013. ISBN: 978-1-62948-233-0 (Hardcover)
2013: ISBN: 978-1-62948-234-7 (eBook)

Public Health Concern: Smoking, Alcohol and Substance Use
Joav Merrick and Ariel Tenenbaum (Editors)
2013. ISBN: 978-1-62948-424-2 (Hardcover)
2013. ISBN: 978-1-62948-430-3 (eBook)

Mental Health from an International Perspective
Joav Merrick, Shoshana Aspler and Mohammed Morad (Editors)
2013. ISBN: 978-1-62948-519-5 (Hardcover)
2013. ISBN: 978-1-62948-520-1 (eBook)

Health Risk Communication
Marijke Lemal and Joav Merrick (Editors)
2012. ISBN: 978-1-62257-544-2 (Hardcover)
2012. ISBN: 978-1-62257-552-7 (eBook)

Adolescence and Chronic Illness. A Public Health Concern
Hatim Omar, Donald E Greydanus, Dilip R Patel and Joav Merrick (Editors)
2012. ISBN: 978-1-60876-628-4 (Hardcover)
2010. ISBN: 978-1-61761-482-8 (eBook)

Child and Adolescent Health Yearbook 2009
Joav Merrick (Editor)
2012. ISBN: 978-1-61668-913-1 (Hardcover)
2012. ISBN: 978-1-62257-095-9 (eBook)

Child and Adolescent Health Yearbook 2010
Joav Merrick (Editor)
2012. ISBN: 978-1-61209-788-6
(Hardcover)
2012. ISBN: 978-1-62417-046-1
(eBook)

Child Health and Human Development Yearbook 2010
Joav Merrick (Editor)
2012. ISBN: 978-1-61209-789-3
(Hardcover)
2012. ISBN: 978-1-62081-721-6
(eBook)

Public Health Yearbook 2010
Joav Merrick (Editor)
2012. ISBN: 978-1-61209-971-2
(Hardcover)
2012. ISBN: 978-1-62417-863-4
(eBook)

Alternative Medicine Yearbook 2010
Joav Merrick (Editor)
2012. ISBN: 978-1-62100-132-4
(Hardcover)
2011. ISBN: 978-1-62100-210-9
(eBook)

The Astonishing Brain and Holistic Consciousness: Neuroscience and Vedanta Perspectives
Vinod D Deshmukh
2012. ISBN: 978-1-61324-295-7

Translational Research for Primary Healthcare
Erica Bell, Gert P Westert and Joav Merrick (Editors)
2012. ISBN: 978-1-61324-647-4
(Hardcover)
2012. ISBN: 978-1-62417-409-4
(eBook)

Our Search for Meaning in Life: Quality of Life Philosophy
Søren Ventegodt and Joav Merrick
2012. ISBN: 978-1-61470-494-2
(Hardcover)
2011. ISBN: 978-1-61470-519-2
(eBook)

Randomized Clinical Trials and Placebo: Can You Trust the Drugs are Working and Safe?
Søren Ventegodt and Joav Merrick
2012. ISBN: 978-1-61470-067-8
(Hardcover)
2011. ISBN: 978-1-61470-151-4
(eBook)

Building Community Capacity: Minority and Immigrant Populations
Rosemary M Caron and Joav Merrick
(Editors)
2012. ISBN: 978-1-62081-022-4
(Hardcover)
2012. ISBN: 978-1-62081-032-3
(eBook)

Applied Public Health: Examining Multifaceted Social or Ecological Problems and Child Maltreatment
John R Lutzker and Joav Merrick
(Editors)
2012. ISBN: 978-1-62081-356-0
(Hardcover)
2012. ISBN: 978-1-62081-388-1
(eBook)

Treatment and Recovery of Eating Disorders
Daniel Stein and Yael Latzer
(Editors)
2012. ISBN: 978-1-61470-259-7
(Hardcover)
2012. ISBN: 978-1-61470-418-8
(eBook)

Human Immunodeficiency Virus (HIV) Research: Social Science Aspects
Hugh Klein and Joav Merrick
(Editors)
2012. ISBN: 978-1-62081-293-8
(Hardcover)
2012. ISBN: 978-1-62081-346-1
(eBook)

AIDS and Tuberculosis: Public Health Aspects
Daniel Chemtob and Joav Merrick
(Editors)
2012. ISBN: 978-1-62081-382-9
(Softcover)
2012. ISBN: 978-1-62081-406-2
(eBook)

Public Health Yearbook 2011
Joav Merrick (Editor)
2012. ISBN: 978-1-62081-433-8
(Hardcover)
2012. ISBN: 978-1-62081-434-5
(eBook)

Alternative Medicine Research Yearbook 2011
Joav Merrick (Editor)
2012. ISBN: 978-1-62081-476-5
(Hardcover)
2012. ISBN: 978-1-62081-477-2
(eBook)

Building Community Capacity: Skills and Principles
Rosemary M Caron and Joav Merrick (Editors)
2012. ISBN: 978-1-61209-331-4 (Hardcover)
2012. ISBN: 978-1-62257-238-0 (eBook)

Textbook on Evidence-Based Holistic Mind-Body Medicine: Basic Principles of Healing in Traditional Hippocratic Medicine
Søren Ventegodt and Joav Merrick
2012. ISBN: 978-1-62257-094-2 (Hardcover)
2012. ISBN: 978-1-62257-172-7 (eBook)

Textbook on Evidence-Based Holistic Mind-Body Medicine: Basic Philosophy and Ethics of Traditional Hippocratic Medicine
Søren Ventegodt and Joav Merrick
2012. ISBN: 978-1-62257-052-2 (Hardcover)
2013. ISBN: 978-1-62257-707-1 (eBook)

Textbook on Evidence-Based Holistic Mind-Body Medicine: Research, Philosophy, Economy and Politics of Traditional Hippocratic Medicine
Søren Ventegodt and Joav Merrick
2012. ISBN: 978-1-62257-140-6 (Hardcover)
2012. ISBN: 978-1-62257-171-0 (eBook)

Behavioral Pediatrics, 3rd Edition
Donald E Greydanus, Dilip R Patel, Helen D Pratt and Joseph L Calles, Jr (Editors)
2011. ISBN: 978-1-60692-702-1 (Hardcover)
2009. ISBN: 978-1-60876-630-7 (eBook)

Rural Child Health: International Aspects
Erica Bell and Joav Merrick (Editors)
2011. ISBN: 978-1-60876-357-3 (Hardcover)
2011. ISBN: 978-1-61324-005-2 (eBook)

Environment, Mood Disorders and Suicide
Teodor T Postolache and Joav Merrick (Editors)
2011. ISBN: 978-1-61668-505-8 (Hardcover)
2011. ISBN: 978-1-62618-340-7 (eBook)

**International Aspects
of Child Abuse and Neglect**
*Howard Dubowitz and Joav Merrick
(Editors)*
2011. ISBN: 978-1-60876-703-8
(Hardcover)
2010. ISBN: 978-1-61122-049-0
(Softcover)
2010. ISBN: 978-1-61122-403-0
(eBook)

**Positive Youth Development:
Evaluation and Future
Directions in a Chinese Context**
*Daniel TL Shek, Hing Keung Ma
and Joav Merrick (Editors)*
2011. ISBN: 978-1-60876-830-1
(Hardcover)
2011. ISBN: 978-1-62100-175-1
(Softcover)
2010. ISBN: 978-1-61209-091-7
(eBook)

**Understanding Eating Disorders:
Integrating Culture,
Psychology and Biology**
*Yael Latzer, Joav Merrick
and Daniel Stein (Editors)*
2011. ISBN: 978-1-61728-298-0
(Hardcover)
2011. ISBN: 978-1-61470-976-3
(Softcover)
2011. ISBN: 978-1-61942-054-0
(eBook)

**Advanced Cancer Pain
and Quality of Life**
*Edward Chow and Joav Merrick
(Editors)*
2011. ISBN: 978-1-61668-207-1
(Hardcover)
2010. ISBN: 978-1-61668-400-6
(eBook)

**Positive Youth Development:
Implementation of a Youth
Program in a Chinese Context**
*Daniel TL Shek, Hing Keung Ma
and Joav Merrick (Editors)*
2011. ISBN: 978-1-61668-230-9

**Social and Cultural Psychiatry
Experience from the
Caribbean Region**
*Hari D Maharajh and Joav Merrick
(Editors)*
2011. ISBN: 978-1-61668-506-5
(Hardcover)
2010. ISBN: 978-1-61728-088-7
(eBook)

**Narratives and Meanings
of Migration**
Julia Mirsky
2011. ISBN: 978-1-61761-103-2
(Hardcover)
2010. ISBN: 978-1-61761-519-1
(eBook)

Self-Management and the Health Care Consumer
Peter William Harvey
2011. ISBN: 978-1-61761-796-6
(Hardcover)
2011. ISBN: 978-1-61122-214-2
(eBook)

Sexology from a Holistic Point of View
Soren Ventegodt and Joav Merrick
2011. ISBN: 978-1-61761-859-8
(Hardcover)
2011. ISBN: 978-1-61122-262-3
(eBook)

Principles of Holistic Psychiatry: A Textbook on Holistic Medicine for Mental Disorders
Soren Ventegodt and Joav Merrick
2011. ISBN: 978-1-61761-940-3
(Hardcover)
2011. ISBN: 978-1-61122-263-0
(eBook)

Clinical Aspects of Psychopharmacology in Childhood and Adolescence
Donald E Greydanus, Joseph L Calles, Jr, Dilip P Patel, Ahsan Nazeer and Joav Merrick (Editors)
2011. ISBN: 978-1-61122-135-0
(Hardcover)
2011. ISBN: 978-1-61122-715-4
(eBook)

Climate Change and Rural Child Health
Erica Bell, Bastian M Seidel and Joav Merrick (Editors)
2011. ISBN: 978-1-61122-640-9
(Hardcover)
2011. ISBN: 978-1-61209-014-6
(eBook)

Rural Medical Education: Practical Strategies
Erica Bell, Craig Zimitat and Joav Merrick (Editors)
2011. ISBN: 978-1-61122-649-2
(Hardcover)
2011. ISBN: 978-1-61209-476-2
(eBook)

Advances in Environmental Health Effects of Toxigenic Mold and Mycotoxins
Ebere Cyril Anyanwu
2011. ISBN: 978-1-60741-953-2

Public Health Yearbook 2009
Joav Merrick (Editor)
2011. ISBN: 978-1-61668-911-7
(Hardcover)
2011. ISBN: 978-1-62417-365-3
(eBook)

**Child Health and Human
Development Yearbook 2009**
Joav Merrick (Editor)
2011. ISBN: 978-1-61668-912-4

**Alternative Medicine
Yearbook 2009**
Joav Merrick (Editor)
2011. ISBN: 978-1-61668-910-0
(Hardcover)
2011. ISBN: 978-1-62081-710-0
(eBook)

**The Dance of Sleeping and Eating
among Adolescents:
Normal and Pathological
Perspectives**
*Yael Latzer and Orna Tzischinsky
(Editors)*
2011. ISBN: 978-1-61209-710-7
(Hardcover)
2011. ISBN: 978-1-62417-366-0
(eBook)

**Drug Abuse in Hong Kong:
Development and Evaluation
of a Prevention Program**
*Daniel TL Shek, Rachel CF Sun
and Joav Merrick (Editors)*
2011. ISBN: 978-1-61324-491-3
(Hardcover)
2011. ISBN: 978-1-62257-232-8
(eBook)

**Chance Action and Therapy:
The Playful Way of Changing**
Uri Wernik
2010. ISBN: 978-1-60876-393-1
(Hardcover)
2011. ISBN: 978-1-61122-987-5
(Softcover)
2011. ISBN: 978-1-61209-874-6
(eBook)

**Bone and Brain Metastases:
Advances in Research
and Treatment**
*Arjun Sahgal, Edward Chow
and Joav Merrick (Editors)*
2010. ISBN: 978-1-61668-365-8
(Hardcover)
2010. ISBN: 978-1-61728-085-6
(eBook)

**Poverty and Children:
A Public Health Concern**
*Alexis Lieberman and Joav Merrick
(Editors)*
2009. ISBN: 978-1-60741-140-6
(Hardcover)
2009. ISBN: 978-1-61470-601-4
(eBook)

**Living on the Edge:
The Mythical, Spiritual,
and Philosophical Roots
of Social Marginality**
Joseph Goodbread
2009. ISBN: 978-1-60741-162-8
(Hardcover)
2013. ISBN: 978-1-61122-986-8
(Softcover)
2011. ISBN: 978-1-61470-192-7
(eBook)

**Alcohol-Related Cognitive
Disorders: Research and
Clinical Perspectives**
*Leo Sher, Isack Kandel
and Joav Merrick (Editors)*
2009. ISBN: 978-1-60741-730-9
(Hardcover)
2009. ISBN: 978-1-60876-623-9
(eBook)

Children and Pain
*Patricia Schofield and Joav Merrick
(Editors)*
2009. ISBN: 978-1-60876-020-6
(Hardcover)
2009. ISBN: 978-1-61728-183-9
(eBook)

**Challenges in Adolescent Health:
An Australian Perspective**
*David Bennett, Susan Towns,
Elizabeth Elliott
and Joav Merrick (Editors)*
2009. ISBN: 978-1-60741-616-6
(Hardcover)
2009. ISBN: 978-1-61668-240-8
(eBook)

**Obesity and Adolescence:
A Public Health Concern**
*Hatim A Omar,
Donald E Greydanus, Dilip R Patel
and Joav Merrick (Editors)*
2009. ISBN: 978-1-60692-821-9
(Hardcover)
2009. ISBN: 978-1-61470-465-2
(eBook)

**Complementary Medicine
Systems: Comparison
and Integration**
Karl W Kratky
2008. ISBN: 978-1-60456-475-4
(Hardcover)
2008. ISBN: 978-1-61122-433-7
(eBook)

Pain in Children and Youth
Patricia Schofield and Joav Merrick
(Editors)
2008. ISBN: 978-1-60456-951-3
(Hardcover)
2008. ISBN: 978-1-61470-496-6
(eBook)

Adolescent Behavior Research: International Perspectives
Joav Merrick and Hatim A Omar
(Editors)
2007. ISBN: 1-60021-649-8

HEALTH AND HUMAN DEVELOPMENT

PSYCHOSOCIAL NEEDS

SUCCESS IN LIFE AND CAREER PLANNING

DANIEL TL SHEK
JANET TY LEUNG
TAK-YAN LEE
AND
JOAV MERRICK
EDITORS

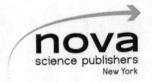

Copyright © 2017 by Nova Science Publishers, Inc.

All rights reserved. No part of this book may be reproduced, stored in a retrieval system or transmitted in any form or by any means: electronic, electrostatic, magnetic, tape, mechanical photocopying, recording or otherwise without the written permission of the Publisher.

We have partnered with Copyright Clearance Center to make it easy for you to obtain permissions to reuse content from this publication. Simply navigate to this publication's page on Nova's website and locate the "Get Permission" button below the title description. This button is linked directly to the title's permission page on copyright.com. Alternatively, you can visit copyright.com and search by title, ISBN, or ISSN.

For further questions about using the service on copyright.com, please contact:
Copyright Clearance Center
Phone: +1-(978) 750-8400   Fax: +1-(978) 750-4470   E-mail: info@copyright.com.

NOTICE TO THE READER

The Publisher has taken reasonable care in the preparation of this book, but makes no expressed or implied warranty of any kind and assumes no responsibility for any errors or omissions. No liability is assumed for incidental or consequential damages in connection with or arising out of information contained in this book. The Publisher shall not be liable for any special, consequential, or exemplary damages resulting, in whole or in part, from the readers' use of, or reliance upon, this material. Any parts of this book based on government reports are so indicated and copyright is claimed for those parts to the extent applicable to compilations of such works.

Independent verification should be sought for any data, advice or recommendations contained in this book. In addition, no responsibility is assumed by the publisher for any injury and/or damage to persons or property arising from any methods, products, instructions, ideas or otherwise contained in this publication.

This publication is designed to provide accurate and authoritative information with regard to the subject matter covered herein. It is sold with the clear understanding that the Publisher is not engaged in rendering legal or any other professional services. If legal or any other expert assistance is required, the services of a competent person should be sought. FROM A DECLARATION OF PARTICIPANTS JOINTLY ADOPTED BY A COMMITTEE OF THE AMERICAN BAR ASSOCIATION AND A COMMITTEE OF PUBLISHERS.

Additional color graphics may be available in the e-book version of this book.

Library of Congress Cataloging-in-Publication Data

ISBN: 978-1-53611-951-0

Published by Nova Science Publishers, Inc. † New York

CONTENTS

Introduction   xxv

Chapter 1   Helping young people with greater psychosocial needs   1
Daniel TL Shek, Janet TY Leung, Tak Yan Lee and Joav Merrick

Section one: Life and career   7

Chapter 2   What we learned from the insiders: Evaluation of a community-based positive youth development program   9
Cecilia MS Ma, Daniel TL Shek, Moon YM Law and Jackie WL Law

Chapter 3   Promotion of positive youth development through a horticultural therapy program   29
Cecilia MS Ma, Daniel TL Shek and Moon YM Law

Chapter 4   Success factors of a community-based positive youth development program   47
Ben Law and Daniel TL Shek

Chapter 5	Identification of success factors of the community-based adolescent project *Ben Law and Daniel TL Shek*	69
Chapter 6	Factors contributing to the success in life and career *Janet TY Leung and Daniel TL Shek*	97
Chapter 7	Perceived benefits of a life and career development program *Janet TY Leung and Daniel TL Shek*	121
Chapter 8	Evaluation of a positive youth development program for low-achieving students *Janet TY Leung and Daniel TL Shek*	145
Chapter 9	Did students apply what they had learned from a positive youth development program in their real-life situations? *Tak Yan Lee, Andrew YT Low and Anthy LY Ngai*	169
Chapter 10	Does students' academic ability make a difference in the learning outcomes of a positive youth development program in Hong Kong? *Tak Yan Lee, Andrew YT Low, Jerf Yeung and Yuki X Jin*	195
Chapter 11	The experiences of early adolescents after joining a positive youth development program *Andrew YT Low, Tak Yan Lee and Roger KL Lau*	209
Section two: Acknowledgments		229
Chapter 12	About the editors	231
Chapter 13	About the Department of Applied Social Sciences, The Hong Kong Polytechnic University, Hunghom, Hong Kong	235

Chapter 14	About the National Institute of Child Health and Human Development in Israel	**239**
Chapter 15	About the book series "Health and human development"	**245**
Section three: Index		**251**
Index		**253**

INTRODUCTION

In: Psychosocial Needs
Editors: Daniel TL Shek et al.

ISBN: 978-1-53611-951-0
© 2017 Nova Science Publishers, Inc.

Chapter 1

HELPING YOUNG PEOPLE WITH GREATER PSYCHOSOCIAL NEEDS

Daniel TL Shek[1-5],*, PhD, FHKPS, BBS, SBS, JP, Janet TY Leung[1], PhD, Tak Yan Lee[6], PhD and Joav Merrick[5,7-10], MD, MMedSci, DMSc

[1]Department of Applied Social Sciences, The Hong Kong Polytechnic University, Hong Kong, PR China
[2]Centre for Innovative Programmes for Adolescents and Families, The Hong Kong Polytechnic University, Hong Kong, PR China
[3]Department of Social Work, East China Normal University, Shanghai, PR China
[4]Kiang Wu Nursing College of Macau, Macau, PR China
[5]Division of Adolescent Medicine, Department of Pediatrics, Kentucky Children's Hospital, University of Kentucky College of Medicine, Lexington, Kentucky, US
[6]Department of Applied Social Sciences, City University of Hong Kong, Hong Kong, PR China

---

* Correspondence: Daniel TL Shek, PhD, FHKPS, BBS, SBS, JP, Associate Vice President (Undergraduate Programme) and Chair Professor of Applied Social Sciences, Department of Applied Social Sciences, The Hong Kong Polytechnic University, Hunghom, Hong Kong, PR China. E-mail: daniel.shek@polyu.edu.hk.

[7]National Institute of Child Health and Human Development,
Jerusalem, Israel
[8] Health Services, Division for Intellectual and Developmental
Disabilities, Ministry of Social Affairs and Social Services,
Jerusalem, Israel
[9]Division of Pediatrics,
Hadassah Hebrew University Medical Center, Mt Scopus Campus,
Jerusalem, Israel and
[10]Center for Healthy Development, School of Public Health,
Georgia State University, Atlanta, Georgia, US

With adolescence childhood is finished and the teen may experiment with dating, smoking and drinking and they may make important decisions without parental knowledge. They may also engage in risky behavior which may pose threats to their well-being and successful transition to adulthood. We can then ask how we can prevent adolescent risk behavior. Traditionally, prevention scientists proposed three forms of prevention. Primarily, tertiary prevention attempts to reduce the harmful consequences of risk behavior, such as treatment of risk behavior (e.g., mental disorders or substance abuse). For some problem behavior which has already occurred, a better approach is to identify those who are "at-risk" as early as possible (i.e., secondary prevention). For example, youth workers may identify those who have suicidal ideation and intervene as early as possible so that they will not harm themselves. In this book we assess whether a community-based program in Hong Kong was effective in promoting adolescent development and explore what factors were associated with the program effects. It is our modest wish that the studies included in this book can help to reveal the successful experience of the project and provide some pointers for the development of programs for adolescents with greater psychosocial needs.

INTRODUCTION

With maturation in different domains, adolescents begin to experiment things which they do not dare to do during childhood. For example, they may experiment dating, smoking and drinking, and they may make important decisions without parental knowledge. They may also engage in risk behavior which may pose threats to their well-being and successful transition to adulthood. Roughly speaking, adolescent risk behavior can be categorized into two types. While internalizing risk behavior includes behavior that creates harm for an individual such as suicidal behavior and substance abuse, externalizing behavior refers to some "acting out" behavior of adolescents which affects other people, such as violence and delinquent behavior. Statistics show that there is an increase in risk behavior in young people throughout the world.

How can we prevent adolescent risk behavior? Traditionally, prevention scientists proposed three forms of prevention. Primarily, tertiary prevention attempts to reduce the harmful consequences of risk behavior, such as treatment of risk behavior (e.g., mental disorders or substance abuse). For some problem behavior which has already occurred, a better approach is to identify those who are "at-risk" as early as possible (i.e., secondary prevention). For example, youth workers may identify those who have suicidal ideation and intervene as early as possible so that they will not harm themselves. Of course, it would be ideal if we could slow down or even eliminate the occurrence of risk behavior by reinforcing the protective factors and weakening the risk factors. This is what primary prevention attempts to do.

As far as "saving lives" is concerned, secondary prevention and primary prevention are far better than tertiary prevention because they can minimize harms created. Nevertheless, the effort put in primary prevention and secondary prevention is far less than the resources devoted to tertiary prevention. With specific reference to secondary prevention, several points should be considered. First, although there are different approaches to secondary prevention, programs that attempt to promote psychosocial competence of the clients are important. The basic argument is that by promoting adolescent psychosocial competence, risk behavior will not take place easily. Second, there is a quest for evidence-based programs that can identify at-risk adolescents as early as possible. Third, workers should understand the factors are conducive to the success of secondary prevention programs instead of only focusing on the program outcomes.

In a comprehensive review of youth prevention programs in the global context, Catalano et al. (1) showed that although there were effective programs, there was only one effective program in different Chinese communities – the Project P.A.T.H.S. in Hong Kong. The Project P.A.T.H.S. is a multi-year positive youth development program with two tiers of programs. For the Tier 1 Programs, they are designed for junior secondary school students irrespective of their risk status. On the other hand, Tier 2 Programs are designed by school social workers in collaboration with teachers in the schools to meet the needs of students with greater psychosocial needs. In some sense, Tier 2 Programs can be regarded as secondary prevention programs which attempt to help adolescents with greater psychosocial needs. Previous studies showed that four types of Tier 2 Programs were commonly conducted, including programs with adventure-based counseling (ABC) elements, programs with community services, programs with ABC and community services elements, and programs with other modes of intervention (e.g., stress management and parent education programs).

Previous evaluation studies have shown that the Tier 2 Programs in Project P.A.T.H.S. were well-received by the program participants. In the context of a positive youth development program, Shek and Lee (2) showed that the program participants (N = 60,241) generally had positive views about the program, workers and perceived benefits of the program. For example, roughly nine-tenths of the students were satisfied with the program and the workers and roughly eight-tenths of the students perceived that the program was able to promote their holistic development.

In the Extension Phase of the project, the project was implemented for another cycle. For the Tier 2 Program, evaluation findings also showed that the Tier 2 Program was well-received by the program participants. Based on the responses of 153,761 respondents, Shek and Sun (3) showed that the respondents were generally positive about the program and the instructors. Most important of all, they had positive views of the positive benefits of the program. For example, roughly nine-tenths of the participants reported that they had positive changes after joining the program. Shek and colleagues (4) also reported that the subjective outcome evaluation tool designed for students with greater psychosocial needs possessed good psychometric properties.

In addition to the Initial Phase and Extension Phase, a Community-Based Implementation Phase was launched in 2013 to meet the needs of young people in the community. Subjective outcome evaluation findings are very encouraging. For example, based on the responses of 4,245 students collected in 2015, it was found that the Tier 2 program was well-received in the areas of program, instructors and perceived benefits (5). Besides, an additional subjective evaluation form based on the program implementers was developed. Evaluation findings showed that the implementers (N = 375) were generally satisfied with the program, their own performance and perceived effectiveness (6).

While the evaluation findings are very positive, there is a need to look at the different projects in depth. In this book, we have selected some successful cases in the Community-Based Implementation Phase. Through these cases, we will gain more understanding of the factors contributing to the success of the Tier 2 programs. There are several features of the studies included in this special issue. First, the case study approach was adopted to understand the implementation quality and effectiveness of the different Tier 2 programs. By doing so, we can uncover the factors contributing to the success or failure of the programs. Second, focus group interviews were conducted in these studies. While acknowledging the limitations of qualitative research, there are several contributions of focus groups, including its ability to reveal diverse views on a program, easy administration, and the use of group dynamics to facilitate expression of views by the program participants. Actually, the focus group methodology has also been extensively used in the Project P.A.T.H.S. (7). It is our modest wish that the studies included in this book can help to reveal the successful experience of the project and provide some pointers for the development of programs for adolescents with greater psychosocial needs.

ACKNOWLEDGMENTS

The Project P.A.T.H.S. and the preparation for this work were financially supported by The Hong Kong Jockey Club Charities Trust. The chapters in this book are based on papers published in the International Journal on Disability and Human Development 2018;17(3) issue.

REFERENCES

[1] Catalano RF, Fagan AA, Gavin LE, Greenberg MT, Irwin CE, Ross DA, et al. Worldwide application of prevention science in adolescent health. The Lancet 2012;379(9826):1653-64.

[2] Shek DTL, Lee TY. Helping adolescents with greater psychosocial needs: Subjective outcome evaluation based on different cohorts. ScientificWorldJournal 2012;2012:Article ID 694018. DOI: 10.1100/2012/694018.

[3] Shek DTL, Sun RCF. Positive youth development programs for adolescents with greater psychosocial needs: Subjective outcome evaluation over 3 years. J Pediatr Adolesc Gynecol 2014;27:S17-25.

[4] Shek DTL, Ma CMS, Siu AMH. Validation of a subjective outcome evaluation tool for participants in a positive youth development program in Hong Kong. J Pediatr Adolesc Gynecol 2014;27:S26-31.

[5] Shek DTL, Ma CMS, Law MYM, Zhao Z. Evaluation of a community-based positive youth development program for adolescents with greater psychosocial needs: Views of the program participants. Int J Disabil Hum Dev 2017. Epub ahead of print 26 Jan 2017. DOI: 10.1515/ijdhd-2017-7007.

[6] Shek DTL, Leung JTY, Ma CMS, Wu J. Subjective outcome evaluation of the community-based P.A.T.H.S Project: Views of program implementers. Int J Disabil Hum Dev 2017. Epub ahead of print 26 Jan 2017. DOI: 10.1515/ijdhd-2017-7008.

[7] Shek DTL. Programme evaluation in the Chinese cultural context. In: Barbour RS, Morgan DL, eds. A new era of focus group research: Challenges, innovation and practice, 1st ed. Hampshire: Palgrave-McMillian, in press.

Section One: Life and Career

In: Psychosocial Needs
Editors: Daniel TL Shek et al.

ISBN: 978-1-53611-951-0
© 2017 Nova Science Publishers, Inc.

Chapter 2

WHAT WE LEARNED FROM THE INSIDERS: EVALUATION OF A COMMUNITY-BASED POSITIVE YOUTH DEVELOPMENT PROGRAM

Cecilia MS Ma[1], PhD,
Daniel TL Shek[1-5],*, PhD, FHKPS, BBS, SBS, JP,
Moon YM Law[1], MSW, RSW and Jackie WL Law[1], BA

[1]Department of Applied Social Sciences,
The Hong Kong Polytechnic University, Hong Kong, PR China
[2]Centre for Innovative Programmes for Adolescents and Families,
The Hong Kong Polytechnic University, Hong Kong, PR China
[3]Department of Social Work, East China Normal University,
Shanghai, PR China
[4]Kiang Wu Nursing College of Macau, Macau, PR China
[5]Division of Adolescent Medicine, Department of Pediatrics, Kentucky
Children's Hospital, University of Kentucky College of Medicine,
Lexington, Kentucky, US

---

* Correspondence: Daniel TL Shek, PhD, FHKPS, BBS, SBS, JP, Associate Vice President (Undergraduate Programme) and Chair Professor of Applied Social Sciences, Department of Applied Social Sciences, The Hong Kong Polytechnic University, Hunghom, Hong Kong, PR China. E-mail: daniel.shek@polyu.edu.hk.

In this chapter we assess whether a community-based program was effective in promoting adolescents' development and explore what factors were associated with the program effects. A total of 406 junior secondary students (Secondary 1-3) from five schools participated in a positive youth development program across three years (2013-2015). Seven focus group interviews were conducted to collect qualitative data from the program implementers, program participants and their parents/caretakers ($N = 46$). Results showed that the program was effective in promoting adolescents' self-competence, beliefs in the future, problem solving skills and interpersonal relationship. Factors that accounted for these changes included the presence of a positive and supportive atmosphere and the presence of a collaborative and experiential learning environment. This study provides evidence on the positive impact of a positive youth development (PYD) program and helps identify factors that facilitate the implementation of PYD programs.

INTRODUCTION

In the first half of the 2016-17 academic year, 19 students committed suicide in six months' time (1). While such tragedies alarmed Hong Kong and we are mourning over their passing, it is crucial for us to think what young people have to face during their adolescent years and what schools, teachers, parents, and stakeholders could offer in order to promote adolescent development.

Developmentally, adolescence is a challenging period in which individuals face several developmental needs and changes when moving toward adulthood. First, when children enter puberty, the hormones controlling physical development are activated and most children develop primary and secondary sex characteristics. Along with hormonal changes, the development within an individual may give rise to intense experiences of rage, fear, aggression (including those toward oneself), excitement and sexual attraction (2). Inevitably, mood disturbance is brought about by biological changes.

Second, along with the biological changes, adolescents also face cognitive changes. During pre-adolescence, young people struggle to assume control that is previously held by their parents/ caretakers but they are not yet fully capable of striking a balance between their own needs and others' needs. During middle to late adolescence, young people learn to distance themselves and start to align their needs with others' within social reality. In post-adolescence, young people further restructure the sense of self and others, producing a self that is more connected and integrated with the society (3).

Third, from the social perspective, materialistic orientation and egocentrism are commonly regarded as attributes of Hong Kong adolescents, which indeed create a certain negative image of them (4, 5). From the economic perspective, Hong Kong is an international city where adolescents are nurtured with material prosperity. Culturally speaking, Chinese parents' concept of success is equivalent to material possession or social status and such conceptions are imprinted in youngsters' mind. Taking family structure into consideration, a declining trend of the average household size from 3.9 in 1981 to 2.9 in 2015 was observed (6, 7). To a certain extent, a smaller family size may contribute to egocentrism in adolescents.

Lastly, for the adolescents who are receiving schooling, most of them feel stressed when their parents strongly emphasize high academic achievement. For those who are going to join the labor force, they may also live under pressure when job-hunting gets tough, which would, in turn, lead to a loss of hope, low self-esteem, and a decrease in overall life satisfaction (8).

The abovementioned challenges increase tension and negativity within adolescents. Indeed, adolescents can develop in a healthy manner when they receive support from adults and are equipped with the skills required to cope with these developmental challenges (9). Recently, the positive youth development approach emphasized individuals' assets and strengths, such as intrapersonal and interpersonal qualities (10). Prior research demonstrated the effectiveness of this program in Western (11,12) and Chinese (13) contexts. However, few studies have examined the perception and benefits of the youth development programs from the perspectives of parents and caregivers. Multiple perspectives for studying the impact of youth programs are important in understanding the outcomes of the program and improving the rigor of research in intervention contexts. As such, this study attempted to fill this research gap with particular reference to whether the positive youth development program designed under the community-based P.A.T.H.S. Project has achieved the outcomes in the target recipients.

To help adolescents develop in a holistic manner, The Hong Kong Jockey Club Charities Trust initiated a project entitled "P.A.T.H.S. to Adulthood: A Jockey Club Youth Enhancement Scheme" (Project P.A.T.H.S.) in 2004. A two-tier positive youth development program was designed and has been implemented for junior secondary school students in Hong Kong since 2005. The Tier 1 programs are universal positive youth development programs whereas the Tier 2 programs are selective programs for students with greater psychosocial needs (13,14). The Tier 2 programs of the Project P.A.T.H.S. are mainly out-of-school programs that allow students to step outside their comfort zone, to safely explore independence, peer relationships, and leadership, and to form long-lasting relationships with adults outside their families (15).

The Tier 2 programs that students join are classified as providing opportunities for prosocial involvement as the activities allow them to actively participate, make a positive contribution and experience positive social exchanges (13). These programs also provide participants with opportunities to develop personal abilities and skills, and hopefully these would enable adolescents to be more confident and capable of tackling difficulties when they develop life goals with hope, optimism, and better problem-focused coping skills. To date, studies of positive youth development programs are mostly quantitative (16,17). Researchers argued for the importance of adopting a qualitative approach to study the effectiveness of positive youth development programs (18,19). This method allows for a better understanding of the impacts and changes in youths after their participation in such programs (20) and it has been used in other contexts, such as community substance abuse treatments (21) and after-school programs for disadvantaged girls (22). Through active listening and good preparation for the interviews, researchers serve as "miners" to understand the target respondents' real world (23,24), which may sometimes be difficult to capture using the quantitative method.

Given the paucity of qualitative research studies examining the impact of positive youth development programs, this study utilized focus group interviews to assess the outcomes of a community-based youth program based on the perceptions of program implementers, program participants, and their parents/caretakers. In particular, we explored whether the program was effective in promoting adolescents' development. Besides, we identified factors that might contribute to the possible changes in the program participants.

OUR STUDY

A total of 406 junior secondary school students (Secondary 1-3, equivalent to Grade 7-9) from five schools participated in the Tier 2 programs across three years (2013: $N = 131$; 2014: $N = 145$; 2015: $N = 130$, Table 1). Program implementers (social workers and class teachers) conducted a total of 261 sessions (total number of hours: 726.5) over the past three years.

Table 1. Background information of the program implementers, program participants, and their parents/caretakers

	2013	2014	2015
Total number of schools	5	5	5
Total number of program participants	131	145	130
Secondary 1	*85*	*90*	*130*
Secondary 2	*30*	*30*	*-*
Secondary 3	*16*	*25*	*-*
Total number of parents of program participants	80	73	59
Secondary 1	*47*	*52*	*59*
Secondary 2	*20*	*20*	*-*
Secondary 3	*13*	*1*	*-*
Total number of program implementers	12	11	9

Table 2 presents different outside school activities/sessions implemented across junior secondary years. In general, students were introduced to different outdoor activities, such as hiking, leadership camps and volunteer service, which focused on developing their problem-solving and interpersonal skills. Through the integration of the adventure-based learning components and the provision of active learning opportunities, students realized their full potential and achieved positive changes in their life.

Table 2. Background information on the Tier 2 programs

Programs conducted		2013	2014	2015
Secondary 1	Opening ceremony, adventure training camp, volunteer training workshops, volunteer service in Hong Kong, volunteer service in rural area in China, inter-school parent-child activities and award presentation ceremony	58 sessions (in total 173 hours)	49 sessions (in total 145 hours)	78 sessions (in total 213.5 hours)
Secondary 2	Opening ceremony, adventure training camp, inauguration ceremony of volunteer team, volunteer service in Hong Kong and closing ceremony	20 sessions (in total 51 hours)	19 sessions (in total 44 hours)	-
Secondary 3	Opening ceremony, adventure training camp, volunteer training workshops, volunteer service in Hong Kong, inter-school parent-child activities and award presentation ceremony	16 sessions (in total 48 hours)	21 sessions (in total 52 hours)	-

In this study, focus group interviews were conducted to assess the program outcomes based on the impressions of multiple sources (program implementers, program participants and the parents/caretakers of the participants, see Table 3). Three semi-structured interview guides were designed: one for program implementers (see Table 4), one for program participants (see Table 5) and one for program participants' parents/caretakers (see Table 6). The interview guides included questions related to their perceptions (e.g., did you notice any changes about yourself (your students/child) after participating in this program?), the impact (e.g., do you think this program has strengthened your (your students'/child's) self-competence?), and overall impression of the program (e.g., how would you describe your (your students'/child's) experiences after participating in this program?). The interviews were conducted by the first and third authors, who had been teaching for over ten years and practiced in social work for more than ten years, respectively. Both conducted more than 50 interviews in the past five years.

Table 3. Background information of the focus group interviews

	No. of waves	Interview period	Participants
Focus group 1	Wave 1	October 2013	6 social workers
Focus group 2		January 2014	10 program participants
Focus group 3	Wave 2	June 2014	7 program participants
Focus group 4			4 parents
Focus group 5			2 school teachers
Focus group 6	Wave 3	July 2015	10 program participants
Focus group 7			7 parents

Note: Each interview was completed in around 60 minutes.

Table 4. A sample of the interview questions (Program implementers' version)

Evaluation of the General Effectiveness of the Program
1. Do you feel that the program is beneficial to the development of the adolescents?
2. Have you noticed any changes in the students after participating in the program? If yes, what are the changes?
3. What do you think are the factors that have caused these changes?
4. If you have not noticed any changes in students, what do you think are the factors that hinder the possible changes?
Evaluation of the Specific Effectiveness of the Program
1. Do you think that the program can develop students' self-confidence or ability to face the future?
2. Do you think that the program can foster students' abilities in different areas, such as spirituality, bonding with family, teachers and peers, compassion for others, a sense of responsibility to the society, family, teachers and peers?

Table 5. A sample of the interview questions (Students' version)

Evaluation of the General Effectiveness of the Program
1. Do you feel that the program is beneficial to your personal development?
2. Have you noticed any changes after participating in the program? If yes, what are the changes?
3. What do you think are the factors that have caused these changes?
4. If you have not noticed any changes, what do you think are the factors that hinder the possible changes?
Evaluation of the Specific Effectiveness of the Program
1. Do you think that the program can develop your self-confidence or ability to face the future?
2. Do you think that the program can foster your abilities in different areas, such as spirituality, bonding with family, teachers and peers, compassion for others, a sense of responsibility to the society, family, teachers and peers?

Purposive sampling of the interviewees was adopted for choosing program implementers (25). The engagement of multiple key informants allowed capturing relevant issues and aspects of the program perceived by different stakeholders (26). Before the semi-structured interviews were conducted, all participants had been asked to sign an informed consent form. Ethical approval was given by the university review board. Seven focus group interviews with a total of 46 participants were conducted between October 2013 and July 2015. Each interview lasted for around 60 minutes (see Table 3).

All interviews were conducted in Cantonese and were recorded using a portable audio recorder. The data were transcribed in verbatim and thematically analyzed. Codes and themes were identified by using constant comparative method (27), the method of analytic induction (25), and principles of grounded theory (open, thematic coding and constant comparison) (28). Member checking and peer-debriefing were used to ensure the trustworthiness of the findings. Emerging codes were discussed using themes relevant to the positive youth development literature (10, 29). Finally, a consensus was reached among the three co-authors (Cecilia Ma, Jackie Law, and Moon Law).

Table 6. A sample of the interview questions (Parents' version)

Evaluation of the General Effectiveness of the Program
1. Do you feel that the program is beneficial to the development of the adolescents?
2. Have you noticed any changes in your child after participating in the program? If yes, what are the changes?
3. What do you think are the factors that have caused these changes?
4. If you have not noticed any changes in your child, what do you think are the factors that hinder the possible changes?
Evaluation of the Specific Effectiveness of the Program
1. Do you think that the program can develop your child's self-confidence or ability to face the future?
2. Do you think that the program can foster your child's abilities in different areas, such as spirituality, bonding with family, teachers and peers, compassion for others, a sense of responsibility to the society, family, teachers and peers?

FINDINGS

In terms of intrapersonal qualities, students reported that after the program, they were more confident about themselves. The following narratives illustrated this theme:

"At the beginning of the task, I didn't think I could make it happen. Interestingly, when I started doing it bit by bit, I got to know myself more. Now, I believe I can make things happen whenever I am confident." (A student from Focus Group 3, Wave 2, 2014)

"I am more confident than before... Many of my classmates and I were shy about speaking in front of a group of people until the day we went to the elderly center. We had to sing a song in front of the elderly." (A student from Focus Group 6, Wave 3, 2015)

The most common benefits that were mentioned in several focus group interviews were participants' beliefs in the future. Many of them commented that they learned to be more optimistic and believe that failure can be overcome.

"We suffered a setback when we first held the fundraising event. In the first few days, we only collected a hundred bucks and our morale was low. But we didn't give up. We encouraged each other and decided to ask our friends to call us. Then, our morale soared as the funds, from a hundred to two hundred and then to four hundred and so on. I valued the transition from failure to success. I developed a sense of achievement when I realized that I could successfully cope with the difficulty ahead of me." (A student from Focus Group 3, Wave 2, 2014)

"Throughout the activities, I learned that when I faced a challenge or difficulty, I could not give up right away but give it a try. In future, I will apply this thinking to my studies. For example, when I see a long article and don't want to read, I would make an effort to read it. I believe if I can make it, I will gain a great sense of achievement." (A student from Focus Group 2, Wave 1, 2014)

Another major theme raised by the interviewees was an improvement of the program participants' interpersonal and social skills. The participants described the importance of effective communications and expressed the value of collaborations with others.

"I think my communications skills improved. At the beginning, we didn't know each other and were too shy to speak to each other. Since we formed a group, we first had to know every member's name, and then we had to name our group and make up our own pose. To be perfect, we had to have very good communications." (A student from Focus Group 6, Wave 3, 2015)

'Use throughout this year, I've learned that sometimes I can't solve a problem on my own but I can get some classmates to face and solve the challenges together." (A student from Focus Group 3, Wave 2, 2014)

One of the notable changes reported by the teachers and parents/caretakers was an improvement of social skills. They described that the participants began to realize the importance of building positive relationships with others, increased awareness of the issues around them and learned to express their concerns to others, even to strangers.

"Last time when we visited an elderly man, who was living alone, we waited for almost two minutes at the door. It turned out that he walked slowly from his bed whereas it may just take us two to three seconds. I learned that we have to be patient with the elderly and have more understanding. We should never think that they are useless." (A student from Focus Group 2, Wave 1, 2014)

"I learned to be punctual after visiting the elderly center. It was a cold day when we visited them. Old people are particularly vulnerable to the flu. So I don't want them to fall sick when they were expecting us. That's why we have to be punctual." (A student from Focus Group 6, Wave 3, 2015)

Teachers' and parents' feedback in the focus group interviews were very encouraging in the sense that they recognized the positive changes in students.

"My daughter had no sense of hierarchy. She always called me and her brother 'meow meow' like a cat. But after she joined this program, she seems to have some respect for authority. She no longer calls me 'meow meow' but mom. She has some respect for me after all." (A parent from Focus Group 7, Wave 3, 2015).

When asked what would be the driving force to help them tackle the difficulties in the activities and finally lead to having positive changes in them, one of the students said,

"Encouragement from people around me is a driving force to overcome the difficulties." (A student from Focus Group 3, Wave 2, 2014)

Students reported that the program created an atmosphere that allowed them to reflect on themselves. This new environment encouraged students to work with others and realized that they were dependent on each other. They learned the importance of creating a positive, mutually understanding, respectful, peer-supporting, and cooperative atmosphere.

"One thing that was very good on this trip to Qingyuan is that they shared a room with a classmate. It's not easy to share a room. No matter whether you like that classmate or not, you would still have to share with him. As they spent time together, he would have learned some skills anyway. It is not possible to just leave the other one alone. And the students were from different schools. This helped sharpen their communication skills." (A parent from Focus Group 4, Wave 2, 2014)

"We walked in pairs on a mountain in the dark one night, with one having his eyes blindfolded. My teammate and I had to trust in each other very much; otherwise, we might have fallen off the mountain. We were dependent on each other so we had to trust each other." (A student from Focus Group 2, Wave 1, 2014)

Sometimes, the smiles or feedback from the service recipients would also be the driving force for the young people:

"It's very encouraging when I see the elderly having a big smile after we taught them handicrafts. It feels good when I help people." (A student from Focus Group 2, Wave 1, 2014)

A final observation from the teachers and social workers is that Tier 2 programs provided a unique context out of the traditional classroom where the ideology of teachers' and students' roles prevailed. The Tier 2 programs, which were usually held out of the classroom, allowed the students to learn through experience and the teachers to not only focus on students' academics but their whole-person development. Through the experiential learning programs, the teachers reckoned that this type of learning opens up an opportunity for them to understand their students and to interact with the students in a friendly manner.

"The kids behaved very differently inside and outside the classroom. Inside the classroom, no matter how many times I asked them questions, they seldom responded. But now, outside the classroom, a kid came and asked me if I needed a hat because it was a hot and sunny day. Last time when we paid a visit to an elderly center, I saw them having a good chat with the elderly. They were very curious and asked the elderly a lot of questions about their lives like their everyday life or the funny things of keeping a dog. Is it our education system that suppresses our kids' curiosity or motivation in school? They seemed weird in the class but they are active and energetic outside the school. Indeed, I find them lovelier outside the school." (A teacher from Focus Group 5, Wave 2, 2014)

"We know that adolescents need recognition and the sense of achievement. When we designed the programs, we allowed the students to gradually take up more responsibilities. We also allowed them to make mistakes. We did not put 'discipline' a high priority, which was different from the classroom setting. So, during the process, the kids were more willing to step outside their comfort zone and try new things. What's important is how we coach them. In fact, their mistakes are the opportunities for us to start the conversation with them and allow them to stay with us with a new perspective on us." (A social worker from Focus Group 1, Wave 1, 2013)

DISCUSSION

Adolescents are facing various challenges, both internally and externally, every day. Increasingly the communities are recognizing the need for youth development programs that concentrate on early prevention and identifying adolescents' needs and strengths. Positive youth development programs are launched to empower the adolescents to tackle the difficulties they face. The purpose of the present study was to explore how a community-based positive youth program helped adolescents to promote their development based on the perceptions from multiple sources. We sought to fill the research gap by assessing whether the program was effective in promoting adolescents' development and what were the factors contributing to these possible changes.

The results showed many positive impacts in the present youth development program. For example, program participants learned to understand themselves more, became more confident about their competence and were more optimistic about the future. They recognized the importance of persistence and the power of support when facing challenges. These findings confirm the notion of positive youth development about the presence of adults' support and caring environment to develop adolescents' strengths and potential (30). Consistent with physical activity studies, students who participated in structured after-school activities, reported positive effects in their psychosocial and behavioral outcomes, such as increased sense of social responsibility, better social relationships and improved competencies (11, 31).

Furthermore, key informants (program implementers and parents/caretakers) noted that the students gained an increased awareness of others and strengthened their sense of community and responsibility. These changes can be viewed as "sensitive" indicators that identify the youth development outcomes after their participation in a positive youth development program (32). Previous studies showed that the lack of identity, feelings of powerlessness and poor social connectedness are common risks faced by adolescents (33). Findings in this study indicated that the program was successful in enhancing students' developmental qualities (e.g., feelings of competency, positive self-perceptions and increased optimism) and establishing a positive social climate. This social context allows them to feel positive about themselves, develop a sense of empowerment and competence, and perceive a supportive atmosphere. The qualitative data indicated that this learning experience of the students provided a social context which required the students to improve social skills (e.g., team building, conflict management, and cooperation). Indeed, these skills need to be taught within supportive and caring social environments (34, 35). Findings of the present study suggest that a warm and empowering atmosphere is important in enhancing adolescents' development.

During the focus group interviews, the students shared their experience on the improvements in both intrapersonal and interpersonal aspects. In terms of intrapersonal qualities, the program participants reported increased self-awareness and self-understanding. Such experiences are beneficial to the development of their self-confidence. Program participants became more confident and skillful at communicating with their peers and expressing their thoughts. They learned the importance of cooperation and team-building and recognized self-discipline. They also learned that things could be solved through conflict management. Moreover, they also used these skills and strategies (e.g., conflict management and peer-learning) to handle daily matters. Lastly, the program participants and implementers noted that the period of participation was relatively short and suggested similar programs should be implemented in the senior secondary school years.

One of the strengths of the present study is that it utilized focus group interviews to understand the impact of the youth development program. This approach "provides a useful way for researchers to learn about the world of others" (24) and allows an in-depth examination of a particular phenomenon (32). In particular, the data collected from multiple stakeholders improved the rigor of our findings. The moving out from the academy to the real-world contexts extended the existing literature (36). Lastly, the results from the present study evaluated the impact of the youth program based on the perspectives of multiple sources (i.e., program implementers, program participants and their parents/caretakers).

Focus group is a commonly used method to promote our understanding of a topic among a group of participants. The focus group methodology generates synergy created by the interaction of group members in generating ideas that would be difficult to obtain via individual interviews. However, some limitations of the focus group method should be noted. First, findings of the present study were based solely on Chinese participants. Generalization to other populations should be interpreted with caution. Second, the data were self-reported at one single time point. Other evaluation methods such as in-depth interviews and longitudinal evaluation should be used to examine the achievement of the programs in the long run. Despite the above limitations, the present study has implications for designing and implementing youth programs. It contributes to the literature by extending our understanding of the impact of a PYD program. Given the paucity of rigorous program evaluation data (29), our study can be viewed as a positive response producing a richer line of evidence-based youth program research (37).

Acknowledgments

The Project P.A.T.H.S. and the preparation for this paper are financially supported by The Hong Kong Jockey Club Charities Trust. The authors thank the school social workers of Hong Kong Children and Youth Services for facilitating the evaluation study. This paper is based on an article published in the International Journal on Disability and Human Development 2018;17(3) issue. We thank the participants for joining this study.

REFERENCES

[1] Oriental Daily. Fifty-eight help-seeking cases of students with suicide questions. Hong Kong, 2016. Accessed 2016 Aug 01. URL: http://hk.on.cc/hk/bkn/cnt/news/20160309/bkn-20160309101856429-0309_00822_001.html.

[2] Nixon R. Adolescent angst: 5 facts about the teen brain. New York, 2012. Accessed 2016 Aug 01. URL: http://www.livescience.com/21461-teen-brain-adolescence-facts.html.

[3] LaVoie JC. Identity in adolescence: Issues of theory, structure and transition. J Adolesc 1994;17(1):17-28.

[4] Shek DTL, Ma CMS, Lin L. The Chinese adolescent materialism scale: psychometric properties and normative profiles. Int J Disabil Hum Dev 2014;13(2):285-95.

[5] Shek DTL, Yu L, Siu AMH. The Chinese adolescent egocentrism scale: psychometric properties and normative profiles. Int J Disabil Hum Dev 2014;13(2):297-307.

[6] HK Census and Statistics Department. Hong Kong domestic household projections up to 2041 (Hong Kong Monthly Digest of Statistics January 2013). Hong Kong, 2013. Accessed 2016 Aug 01. URL: http://www.statistics.gov.hk/pub/B71301FB2013XXXXB0100.pdf.

[7] HK Census and Statistics Department. Population and household statistics analysed by district council district 2015. Hong Kong, 2016. Accessed 2016 Aug 01. URL: http://www.statistics.gov.hk/pub/B11303012015AN15B0100.pdf.

[8] Shek DTL, Leung JTY. Adolescent developmental issues in Hong Kong: Phenomena and implications for youth service. In: Shek DTL, Sun RCF, eds. Development and evaluation of positive adolescent training through holistic social programs (PATHS). Singapore: Springer, 2013.1-13.

[9] Roth JL, Brooks-Gunn J. What exactly is a youth development program? Answers from research and practice. Appl Dev Sci 2003;7(2):94-111.

[10] Larson RW, Hansen DM, Moneta G. Differing profiles of developmental experiences across types of organized youth activities. Dev Psychol 2006;42(5):849-63.

[11] Ullrich-French S, Cole AN, Montgomery AK. Evaluation development for a physical activity positive youth development program for girls. Eval Program Plann 2016;55:67-76.

[12] Vella S, Oades L, Crowe T. The role of the coach in facilitating positive youth development: Moving from theory to practice. J Appl Sport Psychol 2011;23(1):33-48.

[13] Shek DTL, Ma HK, Merrick J. Positive youth development: Development of a pioneering program in a Chinese context. London: Freund Publishing House, 2007.

[14] Shek DTL, Ma HK, Sun RCF. A brief overview of adolescent developmental problems in Hong Kong. ScientificWorldJournal 2011;11:2243-56. DOI: 10.1100/2011/896835.
[15] Eccles JS. The development of children ages 6 to 14. Future Child 1999;9(2):30-44.
[16] Anderson-Butcher D, Iachini A, Riley A, Wade-Mdivanian R, Davis J, Amorose AJ. Exploring the impact of a summer sport-based youth development program. Eval Program Plann 2013;37:64-9.
[17] Bowen DJ, Neill JT, Crisp SJ. Wilderness adventure therapy effects on the mental health of youth participants. Eval Program Plann 2016;58:49-59.
[18] Slesnick N, Dashora P, Letcher A, Erdem G, Serovich J. A review of services and interventions for runaway and homeless youth: Moving forward. Child Youth Serv Rev 2009;31(7):732-42.
[19] Padgett DK. Qualitative methods in social work research, 3rd ed. Thousand Oaks, CA: Sage, 2016.
[20] Royse D, Thyer BA, Padgett DK. Program evaluation: An introduction to an evidence-based approach, 6th ed. Singapore: Cengage Learning, 2015.
[21] Tuchman E, Sarasohn MK. Implementation of an evidence-based modified therapeutic community: Staff and resident perspectives. Eval Program Plann 2011;34(2):105-12.
[22] Hirsch BJ, Roffman JG, Deutsch NL, Flynn CA, Loder TL, Pagano ME. Inner-city youth development organizations: Strengthening programs for adolescent girls. J Early Adolesc 2000;20(2):210-30.
[23] Kvale S. InterViews: An Introduction to Qualitative Research Interviewing. Thousand Oaks, CA: Sage, 1996.
[24] Qu SQ, Dumay J. The qualitative research interview. Qual Res Account Manage 2011;8(3):238-64.
[25] Patton MQ. Qualitative research and evaluation methods, 3rd ed. Thousand Oaks, CA: Sage, 2002.
[26] Mercier C. Participation in stakeholder-based evaluation: A case study. Eval Program Plann 1997;20(4):467-75.
[27] Charmaz K. Constructing grounded theory, 2nd ed. Thousand Oaks, CA: Sage, 2014.
[28] Strauss A, Corbin J. Basics of qualitative research: Procedures and techniques for developing grounded theory, 2nd ed. Thousand Oaks, CA: Sage, 1998.
[29] Catalano RF, Berglund ML, Ryan JA, Lonczak HS, Hawkins JD. Positive youth development in the United States: Research findings on evaluations of positive youth development programs. Prev Treat 2002;5:Article 15. DOI: 10.1037/1522-3736.5.1.515a.
[30] Benson PL, Scales PC, Hamilton SF, Sesma Jr A. Positive youth development: Theory, research, and applications. In: Damon W, Lerner RM, eds. Handbook of child psychology: Theoretical models of human development, 6th ed. New York: Wiley, 2006:894-941.

[31] Weiss MR, Stuntz CP, Bhalla JA, Bolter ND, Price MS. 'More than a game': Impact of The First Tee life skills programme on positive youth development: Project introduction and Year 1 findings. Qual Res Sport Exercise Health 2013;5(2):214-44.

[32] Sandelowski M. Using qualitative methods in intervention studies. Res Nurs Health 1996;19(4):359-64.

[33] DeBate R, Zhang Y, Thompson SH. Changes in commitment to physical activity among 8-to-11-year-old girls participating in a curriculum-based running program. Am J Health Educ 2007;38(5):276-83.

[34] Catalano RF, Berglund ML, Ryan JA, Lonczak HS, Hawkins JD. Positive youth development in the United States: Research findings on evaluations of positive youth development programs. Ann Am Acad Pol Soc Sci 2004;591(1):98-124. DOI: 10.1177/0002716203260102.

[35] Gano-Overway LA, Newton M, Magyar TM, Fry MD, Kim M-S, Guivernau MR. Influence of caring youth sport contexts on efficacy-related beliefs and social behaviors. Dev Psychol 2009;45(2):329-40.

[36] Kurtines WM, Ferrer-Wreder L, Berman SL, Lorente CC, Briones E, Montgomery MJ, et al. Promoting Positive Youth Development The Miami Youth Development Project (YDP). J Adolesc Res 2008;23(3):256-67.

[37] Horn TS. Multiple pathways to knowledge generation: Qualitative and quantitative research approaches in sport and exercise psychology. Qual Res Sport Exercise Health 2011;3(3):291-304.

In: Psychosocial Needs
Editors: Daniel TL Shek et al.

ISBN: 978-1-53611-951-0
© 2017 Nova Science Publishers, Inc.

Chapter 3

PROMOTION OF POSITIVE YOUTH DEVELOPMENT THROUGH A HORTICULTURAL THERAPY PROGRAM

Cecilia MS Ma[1], PhD,
Daniel TL Shek[1-5],*, PhD, FHKPS, BBS, SBS, JP
and Moon YM Law[1], MSW, RSW

[1]Department of Applied Social Sciences, The Hong Kong Polytechnic University, Hong Kong, PR China, [2]Centre for Innovative Programmes for Adolescents and Families, The Hong Kong Polytechnic University, Hong Kong, PR China, [3]Department of Social Work, East China Normal University, Shanghai, PR China, [4]Kiang Wu Nursing College of Macau, Macau, PR China and [5]Division of Adolescent Medicine, Department of Pediatrics, Kentucky Children's Hospital, University of Kentucky college of Medicine, Lexington, Kentucky, US

---

* Correspondence: Daniel TL Shek, PhD, FHKPS, BBS, SBS, JP, Associate Vice President (Undergraduate Programme) and Chair Professor of Applied Social Sciences, Department of Applied Social Sciences, The Hong Kong Polytechnic University, Hunghom, Hong Kong, PR China. E-mail: daniel.shek@polyu.edu.hk.

Most of the horticultural therapy programs have been conducted among individuals with special needs or health-related problems. To better understand how these programs can benefit other service recipients, more research is warranted. The present chapter investigated the impacts of a horticultural therapy program among Chinese secondary school students (Secondary 2) across three years (2013-2015). Both qualitative and quantitative data were collected to explore how the participants perceived such a program. Results showed that over 90% of the students were satisfied with the program and the program implementers. Similar results were shown in the focus group interview data, with participants reporting positive changes in their intra- and interpersonal growth. Findings of the present study extend the literature by demonstrating the beneficial effects of horticultural therapy on adolescents with greater psychosocial needs.

INTRODUCTION

The practice of horticultural therapy (HT) can be dated back to the 1800s when agricultural activities were used to help mental patients. Since the early 1900s and post-war era, horticultural activities have been used for physical rehabilitation in hospital programs (1). Over the past few decades, horticulture, including planting and gardening activities, has been extensively used in psychotherapy and rehabilitation programs in the United States. The establishment of the National Council for Therapy and Rehabilitation through Horticulture (re-named as American Horticultural Therapy Association, AHTA in 1988) further advanced the development of horticultural therapy. After several decades of research and practice, horticulture is regarded as effective in improving cognitive functioning, psychological well-being, as well as social and physical functioning through promoting human-nature interaction (2-4).

Horticultural therapy (HT) was defined by Davis (1) as "a process through which plants, gardening activities, and the innate closeness we all feel toward nature are used as vehicles in professionally conducted programs of therapy and rehabilitation". It is noted that horticulture could be used as a therapeutic modality, which offers numerous advantages in the working process, where people are involved in planning, growing and caring for plants. Horticultural therapy could take effect on individuals by providing meaning to and motivating participants through planting process, producing end products, interaction among participants, and the relationship between humans and environment. It emphasizes the client's engagement in plant-related activities and holds a belief that the active process of horticulture could achieve its therapeutic effects contributing to the designed treatment goals, such as improving mood or attention (2,5,6). Haller (6) summarized that the interaction between humans and plants could bring several advantages, including the encouragement of personal growth and wellness (e.g., the development of positive characteristics like patience and inner peace), mental restoration from fatigue, addressing the innate psychological needs such as providing better living environment, and offering meaning and purpose for establishing a healthy lifestyle. These advantages explained the ways of how horticulture may influence and bring positive changes to individuals.

Many studies have documented the use of horticultural activities in different settings and its benefits to service targets. Haller (7) suggested three main settings using horticultural programs with therapeutic focus: rehabilitation, psychiatric intervention, and long-term care. In rehabilitation programs, horticultural activities are designed for facilitating clients' recovery from an accident or illness, while in psychiatric intervention programs, horticulture activities are planned for managing or healing the illness by increasing tolerance of frustration and managing stress or coping with grief. Regarding long-term care, the activities are designed for maintaining personal functioning such as helping residents relinquish control over their lives through planting. In fact, horticultural activities are widely used in services for elderly with physical disabilities and cognitive impairments such as Alzheimer's disease and dementia (8,9).

In Hong Kong, horticultural and gardening activities are also implemented in nursing homes for the elderly with physical, social, and/or cognitive dysfunction (10,11). Horticultural therapy has been found to be effective in preventing the decline of mental abilities and promoting the overall functioning of the service recipients (12). Besides aged people, it is suggested that horticultural activities could benefit people at different life stages and with special needs (2). For example, a study found that planting activities were effective for children in reducing attention deficit symptoms (13). Another study also found that patients with clinical depression experienced a significant reduction of depressive symptoms after a therapeutic horticulture program. Most of the patients in this study found the program to be meaningful to them and influential for their view about life (14).

Previous horticultural activity programs were mostly implemented among individuals with cognitive or social impairments (9,15), at-risk youth (16,17), people with mental or physical health problems (18,19), and the elderly (20-22). Researchers argued that the therapeutic benefits of horticultural therapy are not limited to any particular ages, genders, cognitive or physical abilities, or cultural groups (23), and regular exposure to nature and green space promotes psychological well-being (13,24,25). Horticultural therapy also promotes quality of life and impacts service recipients positively by reducing stress and enhancing self-esteem and happiness (26-29). In fact, many horticultural programs targeted specific populations including battered women (30) and criminal offenders (16,31). However, it is rare to use horticultural therapy for promoting adolescent development. Theoretically, youth population with developmental needs could benefit from the horticultural activities in promoting their personal growth. There are some existing studies documenting the benefits of planting in an indoor environment for university students (32) and office workers (33).

Recently, horticultural therapy has been introduced in school contexts (34, 35). For example, Robinson and Zajicek (36) found that elementary school students in an experimental group showed significant improvement in their social skills (teamwork) and self-understanding when compared to those in the control group after participating in a one-year school garden program. Similar results were found in other gardening intervention studies (37,38). Horticultural therapy can serve as an ideal context for promoting holistic development among children and adolescents (e.g., 39). Nevertheless, to date, few studies have examined the possible impacts of horticultural therapy among secondary school students by using both qualitative and quantitative approaches. Researchers (35,40) argued the need to combine both qualitative and quantitative methods when studying the outcomes of these school gardening programs. Multiple data collection approaches, including surveys, interviews, and observations, should be used to strengthen the convergent validity of the evidence for effects on the student and school levels (40). Therefore, the present study explored the participants' perception on a horticultural therapy program designed for high school students with greater psychosocial needs. The impacts of the program are discussed in terms of the quantitative and qualitative evaluation outcomes.

OUR STUDY

A total of 59 secondary school students (Secondary 2, equivalent to Grade 8) from two schools participated in the after-school horticultural program in three years ($n = 20$ in 2013; $n = 12$ in 2014; $n = 27$ in 2015). Typically, the HT program was conducted once a week over a 12-week period. Each session lasted for 90-120 minutes. Most of the activities were conducted in classroom except for two sessions, which were outdoor camping and farm visiting (see Table 1). Written consents were obtained from participants and their parents or caretakers prior to the data collection.

Students were invited to complete a subjective outcome evaluation form, which assessed three aspects of the program, namely program quality (8 items), implementer quality (8 items) and perceived program effectiveness (8 items). A total of 43 questionnaires were collected ($n = 15$ in 2013; $n = 10$ in 2014; $n = 18$ in 2015) with a response rate of 73%. A six-point Likert scale was used (1 = Strongly disagree to 6 = Strongly agree). All data were analyzed using SPSS version 23.

In addition, 14 students were recruited to participate in a focus-group interview once they had completed the HT program. Two interviews were conducted in a classroom ($n = 7$ in March 2014; $n = 7$ in March 2015). Participants were asked to describe their experiences in the program and satisfaction with the program. An interview guide was used to assess the participants' perception and overall experiences of the program. Themes related to the perception of the program were categorized and coded by a trained research assistant. To enhance validity, two researchers who were familiar with the program reviewed the emerged themes (41) and reached consensus.

Table 1. Background of the horticultural program

	2013	2014	2015
Period	• After-school period • one session per week (total 12 sessions) • 90-120 minutes per session		
No. of schools	1 school	1 school	2 schools
Program participants	20 students	12 students	27 students
Program implementers	1 horticultural therapist	2 horticultural therapists	2 horticultural therapists
Horticultural activities	• An introduction to the school gardening (e.g., introducing plants and seedlings, basic plant care) • Teaching and practicing gardening techniques and skills: plant propagation (types of separation), cutting (techniques, time, types), planting, and weeding • Introducing different characteristics of foliage and flowering plants • Cooking with herbs, craft activities (e.g., pressed flower photo frame, decorating vase) • Visiting farm gardens		

Table 2. Descriptive statistics among variables across years

	Scale	2013 ($n = 15$) M (SD)	2014 ($n = 10$) M (SD)	2015 ($n = 18$) M (SD)
Content (8 items)	1-6	5.40 (.48)	5.64 (.64)	5.24 (.63)
Effectiveness (8 items)	1-6	5.70 (.62)	5.70 (.62)	5.28 (.58)
Implementers (8 items)	1-6	5.78 (.63)	5.78 (.63)	5.46 (.51)
Total (24 items)	-	5.70 (.61)	5.70 (.61)	5.34 (.53)

FINDINGS

Descriptive statistics are shown in Table 2. Percentages of responses to the three aspects of program evaluation are presented in Tables 3-5. A majority of students were satisfied with the program (100% in 2013; 90% in 2014, 94% in 2015, Table 3) and the program implementers (100% in 2013; 90% in 2014; 95% in 2015, Table 4). Regarding the effectiveness of the program, students reported that the program enhanced their problem solving skills (94% in 2013; 90% in 2014, 100% in 2015, Table 5) and would join similar programs in the future (93% in 2013; 90% in 2014, 78% in 2015, Table 5).

Students' perceptions of the program were assessed based on the focus-group interviews. Several major themes were extracted from the qualitative data. First, students indicated that they perceived the activities positively after participating in the program. They reported positive changes in their attitudes towards nature.

> "After starting to plant, I have changed my values towards plants and flowers. Before, I could only make them die."
>
> "The seeds I planted were different than before; they would not die quickly, and even can germinate. I changed my attitude towards their vitality. They are strong."

Also, students specified that they learned to pay attention and became more patient after participating in the program.

> "I learned to be detail-minded and attentive to what others say. For example, if the sprouts are not properly developed, the plants will not grow well. That's why you need to pay close attention."

Table 3. Frequency of the positive views towards the program

	2013 (n = 15)			2014 (n = 10)				2015 (n = 18)		
	Slightly agree n (%)	Agree n (%)	Strongly agree n (%)	Slightly agree n (%)	Agree n (%)	Strongly agree n (%)		Slightly agree n (%)	Agree n (%)	Strongly agree n (%)
1. The activities were well planned.	1 (7%)	10 (67%)	4 (27%)	1 (10%)	2 (20%)	7 (70%)		4 (22%)	8 (44%)	6 (33%)
2. The quality of the service was high.	-	9 (60%)	6 (40%)	1 (10%)	2 (20%)	7 (70%)		4 (22%)	6 (33%)	8 (44%)
3. The service provided could meet the participants' needs.	-	8 (53%)	7 (47%)	1 (10%)	1 (10%)	8 (80%)		4 (22%)	7 (39%)	7 (39%)
4. The service delivered could achieve the planned objectives.	-	8 (53%)	7 (47%)	1 (10%)	3 (30%)	6 (60%)		3 (17%)	8 (44%)	7 (39%)
5. I could get the service I wanted.	-	7 (47%)	8 (53%)	1 (10%)	2 (20%)	7 (70%)		2 (11%)	8 (44%)	8 (44%)
6. I had much interaction with other participants.	1 (7%)	7 (47%)	7 (47%)	1 (10%)	2 (20%)	7 (70%)		4 (22%)	8 (44%)	6 (33%)
7. I would recommend others who have similar needs to participate in this program.	1 (7%)	8 (53%)	6 (40%)	1 (10%)	1 (10%)	8 (80%)		3 (17%)	6 (33%)	9 (50%)
8. On the whole, I am satisfied with the service.	-	8 (53%)	7 (47%)	1 (10%)	0 (0%)	9 (90%)		1 (6%)	8 (44%)	9 (50%)

Note. All items are measured using a 6-point Likert scale (1 = Strongly disagree to 6 = Strongly agree). Only positive responses (Options 4-6) are shown.

Table 4. Frequency of the positive views towards the program implementers

	2013 (n = 15) Slightly agree n (%)	2013 Agree n (%)	2013 Strongly agree n (%)	2014 (n = 10) Slightly agree n (%)	2014 Agree n (%)	2014 Strongly agree n (%)	2015 (n = 18) Slightly agree n (%)	2015 Agree n (%)	2015 Strongly agree n (%)
1. The worker(s) has professional knowledge.	-	6 (40%)	9 (60%)	1 (10%)	1 (10%)	8 (80%)	1 (6%)	9 (50%)	8 (44%)
2. The worker(s) demonstrated good working skills.	-	5 (33%)	10 (67%)	1 (10%)	1 (10%)	8 (80%)	1 (6%)	9 (50%)	8 (44%)
3. The worker(s) was well prepared for the program.	-	6 (40%)	9 (60%)	1 (10%)	0 (0%)	9 (90%)	2 (11%)	6 (33%)	10 (56%)
4. The worker(s) understood the needs of the participants.	-	7 (47%)	8 (53%)	1 (10%)	0 (0%)	9 (90%)	1 (6%)	5 (28%)	12 (67%)
5. The worker(s) cared about the participants.	1 (7%)	5 (33%)	9 (60%)	1 (10%)	0 (0%)	9 (90%)	0 (0%)	8 (44%)	10 (56%)
6. The worker(s)' attitudes were good.	-	6 (40%)	9 (60%)	1 (10%)	0 (0%)	9 (90%)	0 (0%)	9 (50%)	9 (50%)
7. The worker(s) had much interaction with me.	1 (7%)	6 (40%)	8 (53%)	1 (10%)	0 (0%)	9 (90%)	3 (17%)	7 (39%)	8 (44%)
8. On the whole, I am satisfied with the worker(s)' performance.	-	6 (40%)	9 (60%)	1 (10%)	0 (0%)	9 (90%)	1 (6%)	7 (39%)	10 (56%)

Note. All items are measured using a 6-point Likert scale (1 = Strongly disagree to 6 = Strongly agree). Only positive responses (Options 4-6) are shown.

Table 5. Frequency of the positive views towards the effectiveness of the program

	2013 (n = 15)			2014 (n = 10)			2015 (n = 18)		
	Slightly agree n (%)	Agree n (%)	Strongly agree n (%)	Slightly agree n (%)	Agree n (%)	Strongly agree n (%)	Slightly agree n (%)	Agree n (%)	Strongly agree n (%)
1. The program I joined helped me a lot.	1 (7%)	10 (67%)	4 (27%)	1 (10%)	1 (10%)	8 (80%)	3 (17%)	10 (56%)	5 (28%)
2. The program I joined enhanced my growth.	2 (13%)	9 (60%)	4 (27%)	1 (10%)	0 (0%)	9 (90%)	3 (17%)	8 (44%)	7 (39%)
3. In the future, I would join similar program(s) if needed.	1 (7%)	8 (53%)	6 (40%)	1 (10%)	0 (0%)	9 (90%)	4 (22%)	5 (28%)	9 (50%)
4. I have learnt how to help myself through participating in the program.	1 (7%)	10 (67%)	4 (27%)	1 (10%)	1 (10%)	8 (80%)	3 (17%)	11 (61%)	4 (22%)
5. I have positive change(s) after joining the program.	1 (7%)	9 (60%)	5 (33%)	1 (10%)	0 (0%)	9 (90%)	1 (6%)	9 (50%)	8 (44%)
6. I have learned how to solve my problems through participating in the program.	1 (7%)	10 (67%)	4 (27%)	1 (10%)	1 (10%)	8 (80%)	0 (0%)	11 (61%)	7 (39%)
7. Compare with before joining this program, my behavior has become better.	-	11 (73%)	4 (27%)	1 (10%)	3 (30%)	6 (60%)	3 (18%)	6 (35%)	8 (47%)
8. Those who know me agree that this program has induced positive changes in me.	2 (13%)	8 (53%)	5 (33%)	1 (10%)	2 (20%)	7 (70%)	0 (0%)	10 (59%)	7 (41%)

Note. All items are measured by a 6-point Likert scale (1 = Strongly disagree to 6 = Strongly agree). Only positive responses (Options 4-6) are shown.

A number of students indicated that the program was beneficial to their interpersonal relationships. They commented that their social and communication skills were improved after participating in the program. They learned to respect others and speak confidently.

> "I treat my friends better. I always spoke to my friends in a rude manner, just like ordering them. But now I won't behave like that. I will listen to them first..."
>
> "I have learned to restrain myself... I could not stop talking with my classmates during the class, but now I will listen to what others say before I speak. Because there are other members and everyone should be included in the sharing... I should listen to others, respect others, and I shouldn't occupy all the time by sharing my views."
>
> "I have become more outspoken and talkative. Actually, when I was in a class, I was so passive to answer questions and always asked other classmates to speak first... even when I worked in a group. But now, as we always had group discussions (in the horticulture group), like what we are doing here, my confidence has increased and now I will be the first one to answer the questions in class."
>
> "Sometimes I am a bit impolite to my family... I think my family relationship improved after we grew a plant together. For example, I used to quarrel with my elder sister, but now we cooperate with each other when planting a plant. If my sister watered it again after I just had watered it, the plant would have died."

A number of participants commented that they applied what they learned in the program to other domains.

> *Academic domain:* "I have learned to study hard... It means I must devote more time, and sacrifice time to study."
>
> *Family domain:* "I was seldom aware of my father's health and thought he was okay. But recently he came back home more frequently... I found his diet was bad, and his health was worse than before. I became more worried about him and now will pay more attention to his health."
>
> *Peers domain:* "I have become more patient. In the past, I hated waiting for others... but now I can wait for someone in a subway station

or line up for something… I think it's because I need to water the plants regularly and become more patient after these regular practices…"

DISCUSSION

The purpose of the present study was to explore the perceptions of secondary school students on the school-based horticultural programs. The quantitative findings showed that participants perceived the program positively and felt the program was beneficial to their development. The results are consistent with findings in prior studies (42-44). The majority of the participants indicated that they were benefited from the interaction with nature and others. Perhaps taking care of plants and building new contacts with others outside the classroom promoted individual aspirations and contributed to a meaningful life. These results are consistent with the findings in horticultural therapy literature (45). Nowadays, people usually spend their time indoors, such as playing computer games. This green-based intervention provides an opportunity for participants to interact with others and contact with natural environment (e.g., plants, flowers, leaves, sunlight, and seeds). Interacting with natural environment (e.g., plants, water, and soil) fosters positive emotion, decreases physiological arousal and encourages positive thinking (46). The psychophysiological benefits are further supported in another experimental study (47). The results of the present study are consistent with prior findings (47-49) and underscore the benefits of horticultural programs for promoting psychological well-being and interpersonal relationships in Chinese service recipients.

Also, contact with the natural environment allows the students to leave their stressful everyday life. In particular, these green-based activities provide an alternative way for students to recover from academic-related stress. Different plants such as flowering plants and foliage plants perform a symbolic function as a sign of nature, which serves as a "co-therapist" (50,51) and provides students a relief from the attention fatigue associated with their heavy academic study load (52). The stress relief function is supported by the Stress Recovery Theory (53) and a number of empirical studies (54-56). Our findings showed that the goals of the program were achieved and that the students benefited from this program by engaging in a reflective thinking process to evaluate their strengths and views of themselves.

Besides, the presence of informal learning environment facilitated the interaction among the participants. They learned to work together with respect and caring in order to complete the assigned tasks. Through this interaction, they developed mutual understanding and appreciation of the individual differences among the participants. These social benefits were in line with the prior findings that horticultural activities had positive effects on service recipients in promoting their social competence and interpersonal skills (16, 36, 54).

Several strengths of the present study can be highlighted. First, a psychometrically sound measure was used to evaluate the subjective outcome of the program. Second, the impact of the horticultural program was assessed in a Chinese context, where such research has rarely been conducted. Third, both qualitative and quantitative methods were adopted. However, the present study also has limitations. First, as the present findings were based on a case study, more research is needed to investigate a wider range of green-based activities and participants. Second, as horticultural therapy is "a time-proven practice" (5), future research should adopt longitudinal designs to study the long-term impact of the program. Finally, as the sample size of the present study was small, a large sample should be employed in future studies.

In general, the current study revealed that horticultural programs are feasible and desirable choices for after-school programs designed for students with greater psychosocial needs. The green-based programs promote psychological well-being and facilitate interpersonal skills among Chinese adolescents with greater psychosocial needs. Our findings shed light on evaluation research by showing the potential benefits of horticultural programs. This provides implications for practitioners and educators when designing successful holistic youth programs.

ACKNOWLEDGMENTS

The program presented in the paper was administered under the Project P.A.T.H.S. which was financially supported by The Hong Kong Jockey Club Charities Trust. The authors thank the school social workers of Caritas-Hong Kong for facilitating the evaluation study. This paper is based on an article published in the International Journal on Disability and Human Development 2018;17(3) issue. We thank the participants for joining this study.

REFERENCES

[1] Davis S. Development of the profession of horticultural therapy. In: Simson S, Straus M, eds. Horticulture as therapy: principles and practice. New York: Haworth Press, 1997:3-20.
[2] American Horticultural Therapy Association. Definitions and positions. Seattle, WA: American Horticultural Therapy Association, 2012. Accessed 2016 Aug 01. URL: https://sites.temple.edu/vrasp/files/2016/12/Horticultural-Therapy-.pdf.
[3] Catlin P. Developmental disabilities and horticultural therapy practice. In: Simson S, Straus M, eds. Horticulture as therapy: Principles and practice. New York: Haworth Press, 1997:131-56.
[4] Masuya J, Ota K, Mashida Y. The effect of a horticultural activities program on the psychologic, physical, and cognitive function and quality of life of elderly people living in nursing homes. Int J Nurs Clin Pract 2014;1:Article ID 1:IJNCP-109. DOI: 10.15344/2394-4978/2014/109.
[5] American Horticultural Therapy Association. Horticultural therapy. Seattle, WA: American Horticultural Therapy Association, 2016. Accessed 2016 Aug 01. URL: http://ahta.org/horticultural-therapy.
[6] Haller RL. The framework. In: Haller RL, Kramer CL, eds. Horticultural therapy methods: Marking connections in health care, human service, and community programs. New York: Haworth Press, 2006:1-22.
[7] Haller RL. Vocational, social, and therapeutic programs in horticulture. In: Simson S, Straus M, eds. Horticulture as therapy: Principles and practice. New York: Haworth Press, 1997:43-70.
[8] Connell BR, Sanford JA, Lewis D. Therapeutic effect of an outdoor activity program on nursing home residents with dementia. J Hous Elderly 2007;21(3-4):195-209.

[9] Jarrott SE, Gigliotti CM. Comparing responses to horticultural-based and traditional activities in dementia care programs. Am J Alzheimers Dis Other Demen 2010;25(8):657-65.
[10] Luk KY, Lai KYC, Li CC, Cheung WH, Lam SMR, Li HY, et al. The effect of horticultural activities on agitation in nursing home residents with dementia. Int J Geriatr Psychiatry 2011;26(4):435-6.
[11] Tse MMY. Therapeutic effects of an indoor gardening programme for older people living in nursing homes. J ClinNurs 2010;19:949-58.
[12] D'Andrea S, Batavia M, Sasson N Effect of horticultural therapy on preventing the decline of mental abilities of patients with Alzheimer's type dementia. J TherHortic 2007;18:8-17.
[13] Taylor AF, Kuo FE, Sullivan WC. Coping with ADD: The surprising connection to green play settings. Environ Behav *2001;*33(1):54-77.
[14] Gonzalez MT, Hartig T, Patil GG, Martinsen WE, Kirkevold M. A prospective study of existential issues in therapeutic horticulture for clinical depression. Issues Ment Health Nurs 2011;32(1):73-81.
[15] Jarrott SE, Kwack HR, Relf D. An observational assessment of a dementia-specific horticultural therapy program. Hort Technology 2002;12(3):403-10.
[16] Cammack C, Waliczek TM, Zajicek JM. The green brigade: The psychological effects of a community-based horticultural program on the self-development characteristics of juvenile offenders. Hort Technology 2002;12(1):82-6.
[17] DeAnda D. A qualitative evaluation of a mentor program for at-risk youth: The participants' perspective. Child AdolescSoc Work J 2001;18(2):97-117.
[18] Epstein I. Adventure therapy: A mental health promotion strategy in pediatric oncology. J PediatrOncolNurs 2004; 21(2):103-10.
[19] Grahn P, Stigsdotter UA. Landscape planning and stress. Urban For Urban Green 2003;2(1):1-18.
[20] Burgess CW. Horticulture and its application to the institutionalized elderly. Act Adapt Aging 1989;14(3):51-62.
[21] Detweiler MB, Sharma T, Detweiler JG, Murphy PF, Lane S, Carman J, et al. What is the evidence to support the use of therapeutic gardens for the elderly? Psychiatry Investig 2012;9(2):100-10.
[22] Mooney P, Milstein S. Assessing the benefits of a therapeutic horticultural program for seniors in intermediate care. In: Francis M, Lindsey P, Rice JS, eds. The healing dimensions of people-plant relations. Davis, CA: University California Center Design Research, 1994:173-94.
[23] The Horticultural Therapy Society of New South Wales. Cultivate NSW, 2016. Accessed 2016 Aug 01. URL: http://www.cultivatensw.org.au.
[24] De Vries S, Verheij RA, Groenewegen PP, Spreeuwenberg P. Natural environments—healthy environments? An exploratory analysis of the relationship between greenspace and health. Environ Plan A 2003;35(10):1717-31.
[25] Pretty J, Peacock J, Hine R, Sellens M, South N, Griffin M. Green exercise in the UK countryside: Effects on health and psychological well-being, and implications for policy and planning. J Environ Plann Man 2007;50(2):211-31.

[26] Barton J, Griffin M, Pretty J. Exercise, nature and socially interactive based initiatives improve mood and self-esteem in the clinical population. Perspect Public Health 2012;132(2):89-96.
[27] Collins CC, O'Callaghan AM. The impact of horticultural responsibility on health indicators and quality of life in assisted living. Hort Technology 2008;18(4):611-18.
[28] Rodiek S. Influence of an outdoor garden on mood and stress in older persons. J TherHortic 2002;13:13-21.
[29] Van den berg AE, Clusters MH. Gardening promotes neuroendocrine and affective restoration from stress. J Health Psychol 2011;16:3-11.
[30] Lee S, Kim MS, Suh JK. Effects of horticultural therapy of self-esteem and depression of battered women at a shelter in Korea. ActaHortic 2004;790:139-42.
[31] Mattson RH, Kim E, Marlowe GE, Nicholson JD. Horticultural therapy improves vocational skills, self-esteem, and environmental awareness of criminal offenders in a community corrections setting. Hort Science 2004;39(4):745-840.
[32] Khan AR, Younis A, Riaz A, Abbas MM. Effect of interior plantscaping on indoor academic environment. J Agric Res 2005;43:235-43.
[33] Raanaas RK, Evensen KH, Rich D, Sjøstrøm G, Patil G. Benefits of indoor plants on attention capacity in an office setting. J Environ Psychol 2011;31:99-105.
[34] Alexander J, North M, Hendren DK. Master gardener classroom garden project: An evaluation of the benefits to children. Child Environ 1995;12(2):256-63.
[35] Blair D. The child in the garden: An evaluative review of the benefits of school gardening. J Environ Educ 2009;40(2):15-38.
[36] Robinson CW, Zajicek JM. Growing minds: The effects of a one-year school garden program on six constructs of life skills of elementary school children. Hort Technology 2005;15(3):453-7.
[37] Lineberger SE, Zajicek JM. School gardens: Can a hands-on teaching tool affect students' attitudes and behaviors regarding fruit and vegetables? Hort Technology 2000(3);10:593-7.
[38] Morris JL, Zidenberg-Cherr S. Garden-enhanced nutrition curriculum improves fourth-grade school children's knowledge of nutrition and preferences for some vegetables. J AcadNutr Diet 2002;102(1):91-3.
[39] Bundschu-Mooney E. School garden investigation: Environmental awareness and education. San Rafael, CA: Division of Education, School of Business, Education and Leadership, Dominican University of California 2003:1-39. Accessed 2016 Aug 05. URL: http://files.eric.ed.gov/fulltext/ED480981.pdf.
[40] Ozer EJ. The effects of school gardens on students and schools: Conceptualization and considerations for maximizing health development. Health EducBehav 2007;34(6):846-63.
[41] Lincoln YS, Guba EG. Naturalistic inquiry. Beverly Hills, CA: Sage, 1985.
[42] Shek DTL, Sun RCF. Helping adolescents with greater psychosocial needs: Evaluation of a positive youth development program. ScientificWorldJournal 2008;8:575-85.
[43] Lee TY, Shek, DTL. Positive youth development programs targeting students with greater psychosocial needs: A replication. ScientificWorldJournal 2010;10:261-72.

[44] Shek DTL. Is subjective outcome evaluation related to objective outcome evaluation? Insights from a longitudinal study in Hong Kong. J Pediatr AdolescGynecol 2014;27:50-6.
[45] Hassink J, Elings M, Zweekhorst M, van den Nieuwenhuizen N, Smit A. Care farms in the Netherlands: Attractive empowerment-oriented and strengths-based practices in the community. Health Place 2010;16(3):423-30.
[46] Grahn P, Tenngart Ivarsson C, Stigsdotter UK, Bengtsson IL. Using affordances as a health-promoting tool in a therapeutic garden. In: Ward-Thompson C, Bell S, Aspinall P, eds. Innovative approaches to researching landscape and health. Oxford: Routledge, 2010:116-54.
[47] Kim E, Mattson RH. Stress recovery effects of viewing red-floweringgeraniums. J TherHortic 2002;13:4-12.
[48] Matsuo E. Horticulture helps us to live as human beings: Providing balance and harmony in our behavior and thought and life worth living. ActaHortic 1994;391:19-30.
[49] Söderback I, Söderström M, Schälander E. Horticultural therapy: The 'healing garden' and gardening in rehabilitation measures at Danderyd Hospital Rehabilitation Clinic, Sweden. PediatrRehabil 2004;7(4):245-60.
[50] Berger R, McLeod J. Incorporating nature into therapy: A framework for practice. J SystTher 2006;25(2):80-94.
[51] Clatworthy J, Hinds J, Camic P. Gardening as a mental health intervention: A review.Ment Health Rev J 2013;18(4):214-25.
[52] Kaplan R, Kaplan S. The experience of nature: A psychological perspective. Cambridge, UK: Cambridge University Press, 1989.
[53] Ulrich RS. Aesthetic and affective response to natural environments. In: Altman I, Wohlwill JF, eds. Behavior and the natural environment. New York: Plenum, 1983:85-125.
[54] Kam MCY, Siu AMH. Evaluation of a horticultural activity programme for persons with psychiatric illness. Hong Kong J OccupTher 2010;20(2):80-6.
[55] Park SH, Mattson RH, Kim E. Pain tolerance effects of ornamental plants in a simulated hospital patient room. ActaHortic 2004;639:241-7.
[56] Park SH, Mattson RH. Therapeutic influences of plants in hospital rooms on surgical recovery. Hort Science 2009;44(1):102-5.

In: Psychosocial Needs
Editors: Daniel TL Shek et al.
ISBN: 978-1-53611-951-0
© 2017 Nova Science Publishers, Inc.

Chapter 4

SUCCESS FACTORS OF A COMMUNITY-BASED POSITIVE YOUTH DEVELOPMENT PROGRAM

Ben Law[1,*], *PhD, RSW and*
Daniel TL Shek[2-6], *PhD, FHKPS, BBS, SBS, JP*

[1]Department of Social Work and Social Administration, The University of Hong Kong, Hong Kong, PR China, [2]Department of Applied Social Sciences, The Hong Kong Polytechnic University, Hong Kong, PR China, [3]Centre for Innovative Programmes for Adolescents and Families, The Hong Kong Polytechnic University, Hong Kong, PR China, [4]Department of Social Work, East China Normal University, Shanghai, PR China, [5]Kiang Wu Nursing College of Macau, Macau, PR China and [6]Division of Adolescent Medicine, Department of Pediatrics, Kentucky Children's Hospital, University of Kentucky School of Medicine, Lexington, Kentucky, US

In this chapter we examine the effectiveness of a positive youth development program in Hong Kong, where we conducted two separate focus group interviews with program *participants* and program

---

[*] Correspondence: Ben Law, PhD, Department of Social Work and Social Administration, The University of Hong Kong, Pokfulam Road, Hong Kong, PR China. Email: blaw@hku.hk

implementers as participants. The participants were also asked to complete subjective outcome evaluation questionnaires, and the related findings were used to supplement the findings from the interviews. The findings generally showed that the program had positive impact on the program participants, and its effectiveness was primarily reinforced by four factors. They included 1) active participation of students, 2) good design of the program, 3) good professional skills and techniques of social workers, and 4) active involvement of teachers. In conjunction with the previous studies, this result further support the claim that the community-based Project P.A.T.H.S. is effective in promoting positive development of Chinese adolescents in Hong Kong.

INTRODUCTION

This chapter documents the success of a program in the community-based P.A.T.H.S. Project initiated and financially supported by the Hong Kong Jockey Club Charities Trust. In addition to the Initial Implementation Phase (2005 to 2012), the Extension Phase (2009 to 2016) and the Community-Based Implementation Phase (2013 to 2017) were later evolved from the project. In the Community-Based Implementation Phase, the first batch of the program was launched in January 2013, while the second batch was launched in August 2014.

The Hong Kong Lutheran Social Service (HKLSS) participated in the first batch of programs from January 2013 to December 2015, with the Lutheran School Social Work Unit and Rainbow Lutheran Center participating as the service units. HKLSS implemented the Project P.A.T.H.S. starting from 2005 and had since benefited over 5,000 student participants. Given its long history of implementing the Project P.A.T.H.S., HKLSS gathered valuable experience in project implementation and brought forth the positive effects of the project to the broader community. The service units implemented the programs in three secondary schools in the Sai Kung District of Hong Kong. A secondary school which admits students with higher academic attainment was chosen for the present study.

Table 1. Basic information of the Tier 1 Program in the sampled schools

Banding of the School	Mode of Tier 1 Program	Service Users	No. of hours	Time of Implementation
Band 1	Other mode: • One camp (@ 4 h) • Two workshops (@ 1.5 h) • Three lessons (@ 1 h)	140 Secondary 1 students 160 Secondary 3 students	10 hours	• In-class • After school • Post exam • School holiday

Table 2. Tier 2 Program for secondary 1 students in 2013

Content	Activities
• Introduction to the program • Relationship building • Enhance self-awareness of the participants (personal strengths and weaknesses)	• Workshop (one session)
• Promote knowledge on emotional regulation • Enhance the emotional regulation ability of the participants to create a sense of security and affiliation with their peers and family	• Workshop (one session)
• Improve the social skills of the participants and cultivate their appropriate attitudes toward people to facilitate the establishment of interpersonal and familial relationships • Enhance the self-efficacy of the participants by providing them feedback for their participation in the program	• Volunteer training (two sessions) • Volunteer service (one session)
• Enhance problem solving ability, self-confidence, self-efficacy, and sense of uniqueness of the participants • Improve social skills of the participants and cultivate their appropriate attitudes toward people to facilitate the establishment of interpersonal and familial relationships and to resist undesirable behaviors, such as drug addiction and joining gangs	• Outdoor activities (four sessions)
• Apply social and emotional regulation skills of these participants in practice and conduct parent–child activities to foster parent–child relationships • Recognize the efforts of the participants and encourage them to sustain the changes induced by the program	• Parent–child activities (two sessions) • Celebration ceremony (one session)

The Project P.A.T.H.S. entails two tiers of programs, with the Tier 2 program developed by school social workers targeting young people with greater psychosocial needs. For the Tier 1 Program, a 10-hour core program with various learning modes was adopted in response to the needs of the participating schools (see Table 1). Table 2 highlights the positive youth development constructs involved in the Tier 1 Program. The Tier 2 Program attempted to promote the self-esteem of participants via experiential learning. This program specifically attempted to: 1) enhance self-awareness, emotion regulation, sense of uniqueness, and positive thinking of the participants; 2) promote healthy peer relationship by equipping the participants with the necessary social skills and interpersonal attitudes as well as fostering their exposure; 3) enhance participants' interpersonal skills and accordingly boosts their sense of security in their families; 4) cultivate the sense of direction of the participants via *goal setting* and *solution finding*; and 5) improve self-efficacy of the participants by helping them recognize their own values and abilities. Table 3 illustrates the positive youth development constructs as utilized in the Tier 2 Program. Two separate Tier 2 programs were launched for Secondary 1 students (see Table 2) and Secondary 3 students (see Table 3).

Table 3. Tier 2 Program for secondary 3 students in 2013

Content	Activities
• Introduction to the program • Relationship building • Enhance self-awareness of the participants (personal strengths and weaknesses)	• Workshop (one session)
• Promote knowledge on interpersonal relationships and cultivate appropriate attitudes toward people • Cultivate hobbies, abilities, and self-efficacy of the participants by organizing art workshops and training programs	• Workshop (three sessions)
• Promote knowledge on the consequences of drug abuse and cultivate a healthy social circle to resist temptation from drugs	• Talk
• Enhance problem solving ability, self-confidence, self-efficacy, and sense of uniqueness of the participants • Enhance sense of security and affiliation of the participants by conducting team activities	• Outdoor activities (six sessions)
• Recognize the efforts of the participants and encourage them to sustain the changes induced by the program	• Celebration ceremony (one session)

Self-esteem serves as the key element in the Tier 2 Program as stated in the program goals. In his website, Branden (1) defined self-esteem as the "disposition to experience oneself as being competent to cope with the basic challenges of life and being worthy of happiness". In other words, self-esteem refers to one's confidence in his/her ability to think and perform. Theoretically, success, happiness, and achievement are essential in building self-esteem. Children begin to develop their self-perceptions, including an overall description of their own views and attitudes as they grow up and accumulate life experiences. These experiences, which may either be positive or negative, form the basis on which an individual examines his/her ability and self-worth. This self-assessment process, together with the associated emotional changes, constitutes self-esteem (2).

Borba and Taylor-McMillan (3) suggested that there are five building blocks of self-esteem. The first block is *Security*, which is attained by adolescents' knowledge about what is expected from them, feelings of safety and comfort, and development of a trusting relationship. The second block is *Selfhood*. Adolescents with this quality are endowed with a realistic understanding about oneself and a sense of individuality. The third block is *Affiliation*, where adolescents experience a sense of belonging and acceptance with important others. The fourth building block is *Mission*. Adolescents with mission are motivated and set realistic and achievable goals for themselves, and are eager to undertake whatever consequences of their very own actions. The final block is *Competence*, which is characterized by the adolescents sense of accomplishment (on things they deemed valuable or important) and awareness and acknowledgement of their own strengths and weaknesses.

Given that the competitive education system in Hong Kong can easily bestow "failures" upon the teenagers, the self-image and self-esteem of these individuals must be carefully attended to. One possible way to promote self-esteem is to encourage students to learn from their experiences and reflections by engaging in experiential learning. According to Kolb (4), learners must be willing to participate actively in the learning process and be able to reflect on their learning experiences. He illustrated the learning process in the following four-step model: the learners 1) gather physical experience, 2) use this experience as a basis for observation and reflection, 3) conceptualize and improve their performance based on their previous experiences, and 4) engage in experimentation before entering another learning cycle.

To understand the intervention effect on the program participants, there is a need to conduct systematic evaluation of programs. This study attempted to understand the views of adolescents and social workers after they had joined the Tier 2 Program of the community-based P.A.T.H.S. Project. In particular, this study evaluated the effects of the Project P.A.T.H.S. on service users and explored the factors that motivate the positive development of junior secondary school students in Hong Kong.

OUR STUDY

The three-year community-based Project P.A.T.H.S. was implemented by the Lutheran School Social Work Unit and the Rainbow Lutheran Centre of HKLSS in three secondary schools between academic years 2013 and 2015. All these schools adopted the 10-h Core Tier 1 Program with different participation modes and joined the Tier 2 Program. The Tier 1 Program focused on eight positive youth development constructs, including resilience, social competence, emotional competence, moral competence, self-determination, spirituality, self-efficacy and beliefs in future. After the implementation of the Tier 1 Program, these schools were invited to participate in the Tier 2 Program, which aimed to develop qualities in students, including bonding (with others), resilience, social competence, behavioral competence, self-determination, spirituality, self-efficacy, clear and positive identity, and recognition of positive behavior. Altogether there were 480 students joining the Tier 1 Program.

Two-hundred and eight Secondary 1 (Grade 7) students participated in the Tier 2 Program from 2013 to 2015 (see Table 4). The Tier 2 Program was designed for students to know more about themselves and the needy in the community. Through activities such as psychological quizzes and adventure-based programs, students discovered about their strengths and weaknesses. Program implementers were also trained their goal-setting and emotion regulation skills in these activities. Parents were invited in some Tier 2 programs. They interacted with their children and learned about communication skills at home which could improve the parent–child relationship. Apart from enhancing self-understanding (and family relationship), students were encouraged to explore their community. For instance, program implementers designed activities for students to experience the difficulties of visually-challenged persons in their everyday life, and it was hoped that via experience like such the students could be more considerate to this particular segment of population. Students also received training on interaction and communication skills with elderly people. They were then given opportunities to plan for and participate in a voluntary service with these elders. The program was concluded by a prize ceremony which primarily concerns showing appreciation toward the students for their participation and involvement throughout the program.

In 2015, the program implementers organized an extra program for students coming from the above three schools to participate in a movie-making activity. Students were invited to meet each other in the beginning, and to learn about skills for preparing and making a movie. Finally, a screening event — during which students 'premiered' their own movies and talked about their experience in the course of making such — was organized.

Upon completion of each session, both students and program implementers were given an avenue to opine on the program by filling out a program evaluation form. One school was selected for an in-depth qualitative study to explore the factors conducive to the effectiveness of the program. During the evaluation phase, two separate focus group interviews were conducted with students and social workers. Two students (Secondary 1 and Secondary 2) from the selected school were chosen by social workers to partake in a series of in-depth focus-group interviews and accordingly shared their views on the program. Two social workers were also invited to participate in this interview to weigh in with their observations and experiences while they implemented the program.

The interviewees were told a priori about the purpose of the interview and the principle of confidentiality, and then were asked to provide their informed consent to join the study. A trained research assistant with a master's degree in social work conducted the interview. The interviews with students (took about 40 minutes) and social workers (took about 30 minutes) were administered in June 2015. The focus group interview was audio recorded with interviewees' consents. The students were encouraged to comment on the *content, design, program implementers,* and other aspects of the program, while the social workers were encouraged to share their wisdom in designing and implementing the program in the selected school.

We aggregated the subjective outcome evaluation data from the participants and program implementers (Forms A and C for Tiers 1 and 2 programs for the students, and Forms B and D for Tiers 1 and 2 programs for the program implementers) to form an aggregated picture on the views of different stakeholders on the program, with the collection of both quantitative and qualitative data (5–8). The evaluation results supplemented the findings from the focus group interviews in this study.

Instruments

Two specific, self-constructed, semi-structured interview guides were designed for the focus group interviews (see Appendix A).

Focus group interview with the participating students
The themes of interview questions for the students are outlined as follows:

Table 4. Number of schools, participants and program implementers participated in the Tier 2 Program over three years

	2013	2014	2015
Number of school	3	3	3
Total number of core participants + (parents)	68 (23)	76(28)	64 (0)
S1	68	76	64
S2	/	/	/
S3	/	/	/
Program implementers	6	5	5

- Their opinions on the program activities in which they participated and enjoyed;
- Their self-reports on the changes they experienced and things they learned after joining the program;
- Their views on specific aspects of the program, including its *content, design, attitude*, and *program implementers*; and
- Their general perceptions toward the program.

Focus group interview with the social workers
The themes of interview questions for the social workers are outlined as follows:

- Their views on the Tier 1 program, including its major activities, the observed changes among the students, and the factors that contributed to these changes;
- Their views on the Tier 2 program, including its major activities, the observed changes among the students, and the factors that contribute to such changes; and
- Their general perceptions toward the effectiveness and success of the program.

The audio-recorded interviews were transcribed and checked for accuracy by a research assistant.

FINDINGS

The focus group interviews and the consolidated data from the subjective evaluation reports support the positive effects of the Project P.A.T.H.S. on the participants. According to the reports, students were satisfied with the program (see Table 5). They found the activities, especially those in the adventure camp, interesting and fun. The students also deemed the program implementers friendly and well-prepared (in interacting with students and also teaching about cooperation and communication techniques). Nonetheless, they added that adjustment in difficulty may be warranted for some activities, and that more time should be allowed for these activities. Some students also suggested that the less extroverted participants may be insufficiently attended to by the program implementers and other students. In general, students acknowledged that the program had great impact on them and had positive changes to their lives. More than 80% of them agreed that the program helped them develop their moral competence, team spirit, confidence, interpersonal skills, friendship, communication, and resilience.

The program implementers were overall satisfied with how the program was implemented. Table 6 details the program implementers' evaluation of the program. They found the program, which included various types of activities, effective in promoting multi-dimensional development of students. The program implementers also noted that while some students — thanks to their inexperience with voluntary services — may appear withdrawn at the beginning, they became more proactive and involved as the program went on. Specifically, the implementers noticed a gradual improvement in motivation and cooperativeness among students as they were given more opportunities to work with one another and became more skilled at communicating and cooperating with others over the program. However, the implementers also acknowledged that the program was not without challenges. For instance, they found it difficult to coordinate the schedule of the program to fit into students' timetable. Considering that students' involvement (in the program) is inextricably tied to how the program (or specific activities) appealed to them, some implementers may thus have to 'go the extra mile' to, at the very least, preserve their interest and motivation to do well in the program.

In the focus group interviews, some students described the positive aspects of the program as follows: *"I've had many good memories in the program,"* *"I am happy with my choice to have joined the program,"* *"I like the entire program,"* *"I like all of them,"* *"I give 8 to 9 out of ten to the program."* These positive aspects are summarized and explained in the following.

Table 5. Feedback from participants collected from evaluation forms

	2013 N	Mean	SD	2014 N	Mean	SD	2015 N	Mean	SD	overall N	Mean	SD
Views towards the program	68	5.04	.75	75	4.91	.85	61	4.69	1.17	204	4.88	.94
Views towards the workers	68	5.28	.73	76	5.03	.84	64	4.75	1.26	208	5.02	.98
Perceived effectiveness of the program	66	4.92	.78	74	4.86	.80	58	4.72	1.23	198	4.84	.94

Note: Participants rated from 1 (strongly disagree) to 6 (strongly agree).

Table 6. Feedback from program implementers collected from evaluation forms

	2013 N	Mean	SD	2014 N	Mean	SD	2015 N	Mean	SD	overall N	Mean	SD
Views towards the program	6	5.23	.47	5	5.15	.35	5	5.08	.17	16	5.17	.34
Views towards the workers	6	5.00	.56	5	5.13	.34	5	5.08	.17	16	5.06	.38
Perceived effectiveness of the program	6	5.02	.26	5	5.08	.42	5	5.08	.17	16	5.05	.28

Note: Participants rated from 1 (strongly disagree) to 6 (strongly agree).

First, the students claimed that apart from making new friends, they also managed to strengthen their existing bonds with their other friends who were part of the program. Second, the students appreciated the opportunity to explore new things such as making bread and making videos. The students particularly alluded to two key events that offered them unique experiences. While partaking in the community service event for the elderly, students learned that *"the elderly needs someone to talk to and take care of them,"*, and they also acquired certain know-how on conversing respectfully and effectively with the elderly (i.e., *"to communicate with the elderly,"* and *"specific communication skills, such as not using English to talk with these people.)"* Meanwhile, through the filmmaking event the students managed to pick up certain specific movie-making skills such photography, video-editing, on-field problem-solving, and acting. All in all, via these events the students learned to appreciate the importance of solidarity, team spirit, assertiveness and prosociality. Specifically, they credited these events for helping them learn *"to follow the instructions of directors,"* *"to give their opinions on the topic under discussion,"* and *"to assist others who need help."*

The social workers also noted some positive changes in their students as reflected in the following responses: *"Before joining the program, some students only had a few friends in school and received negative comments from their school teachers. After the program, the school teachers witnessed great improvements in some of their students. The teachers also found that their students turned their weaknesses into strengths after joining the program. The program also improved the students' relationships with the teachers and with other students."* The program also improved their self-esteem, sense of achievement, confidence, interpersonal skills, and relationship of these students with others.

Besides these general positive findings, the focus group interviews and consolidated reports also revealed several factors that contributed to the development of junior secondary schoolers. It is worth noting that there was no negative feedback about the program in any of the interviews.

Active participation of students

A social worker attributed the success of the program to the participation of the students. Apart from their varying extent of participation at the beginning of the program, some students demonstrated a higher motivation to participate than others for several reasons. For instance, those students who came from the grassroots or had limited exposure to outdoor activities would very much value the opportunity to participate in the activities offered by the program, such as camping and community service. Accordingly, these students would understandably expend more efforts in the course of the activities and hence be more likely to derive more enjoyment out of the program. One student was evidently excited during the interview while recounting her experience with the program. Apart from being an active participant when she first joined the program as a Secondary 1 student, she was also appointed as a 'senior officer' to help the fellow junior schoolmates. A social worker also noticed the high degree of participation among some students. Therefore, the success of the program can be partly attributed to the active participation of students.

Good program design

The social workers also emphasized the importance of program design in the success of the program. First, the program adopted activity-based learning. The Tier 2 Program included many activities, such as war games, community service for the elderly, and filmmaking. They argued that innovative and outdoor activities must be organized to encourage student participation. Instead of conventional learning modes such as classroom learning, the social workers subscribed to the idea that the optimal learning mode should entail active participation of students. Needless to say, the students' propensity to participate would very much hinge on how 'appealing' or 'interesting' the activities sounded to them. Since the majority of the student participants had rarely played war games or shot movies before, there was definitely an element of 'freshness' in the program which should heighten students' enthusiasm in the program. One should reasonably expect such an elevated enthusiasm to ultimately translate into a willingness to participate and accordingly develop in the course of the activities.

Teamwork and cooperation were identified as the "main courses" in the activity design instead of the activity content per se. In the adventure camp, the students were required to cook their own meals. In the community service for the elderly, the students were asked to organize some activities with the objective to entertain while also assist the elderly. The students were required to interact with others in these activities, thereby offering them the chance to develop their interpersonal and conflict resolution skills.

An intensive training summer program was also organized to enhance group cohesion. Given that students were freed from their academic schedules and hence had plenty of spare time during their summer vacation, they predictably showed better attendance in the program and a marked improvement in their group cohesion over the summer. The social workers also mentioned that implementing summer events, especially in the Tier 2 Program, could ensure better participation of the students. Given the availability of the students, an intensive training design can be practically implemented. The students may be stipulated to socialize with one another and subsequently discuss matters related to the event as a group — in so doing the students should be endowed with sufficient time to develop group dynamics.

Skills and techniques of social workers

The skills and techniques of social workers also contributed to the success of the program. During different events, the social workers observed some changes in the behaviors and characteristics of students inside and outside school. Most students enjoyed listening to how others perceive them. These students especially enjoyed listening to the comments of people they trust, such as social workers, and these comments helped them solidify their self-images. After completing an event and receiving feedback from social workers, the students were required to attend a debriefing session during which they were expected to reflect upon what they managed to learn about themselves throughout. This should offer an avenue for self-improvement among the students as they were given a chance to know more about themselves. Apart from conducting a group debriefing session, an appreciative culture was also cultivated in the program. Being on the receiving end of appreciation for an improvement can no doubt boost the self-esteem of the recipient. At the end of the debriefing session, the social workers usually heaped praises upon the students for their nice behaviors or improvement and encourage mutual appreciation among the students. In so doing, the social workers endeavored to establish an atmosphere of appreciation within the program, thereby emphasizing the crucial role of appreciation in the success of the program. Although the social workers acknowledged that such an appreciation may appear trivial, for instance, just a tap on one's shoulder as a symbol of showing gratitude, they stressed that such a culture of appreciation could spread within peer groups which ultimately may bring forth certain sustained post-program effects.

Good participation of teachers

The active participation of teachers was also indispensable to the success of the Project P.A.T.H.S. The school mandated that each outdoor activity must involve a teacher, thereby providing teachers with an opportunity to understand their students holistically. These teachers — who normally had a relatively partial, confined understanding of their students (as they might be too fixated upon their *academic* performance only) — may now have the 'golden' opportunity to discover the 'hidden potentials' or talents of their students. The social workers noted that some teachers were surprised upon learning about the positive, unknown sides of their students after joining their students in those outdoor activities within the program. Upon this newfound awareness of the strengths of those students, the teachers should be more capable of offering a more 'customized' and positive feedback which should help nurture their students' self-esteem.

Furthermore, the program appeared to have morphed teachers into another important source of motivation who is now capable of seeing the positives among their students. Before joining the program, the teachers generally perceived their students as having poor academic performance, behavioral and emotional problems, limited social network, and underdeveloped social skills. They soon discarded such a negative appraisal once they identified the positive characteristics of their students during the program. Consequentially, they began to offer positive feedback to their students and encouraged their positive behaviors. Such feedback helped these students establish their confidence and importantly, the willingness to attempt to interact with or relate to others in a different fashion. Therefore, the program can also expand the social network of these students.

DISCUSSION

The present study outlined several factors behind the success of the P.A.T.H.S. Project. The focus group interviews and the consolidated data from the evaluation reports identified that *active participation of students, good program design, good professional skills and techniques of social workers*, and *active involvement of teachers* were the major driving forces behind the success of the program. These findings are consistent with the literature on the pillars of a successful program.

It is crystal clear that a program cannot be considered effective without the *active involvement of the participants*. The social workers overall acknowledged the significant role of students in the success of a program. As a result, it is also noteworthy to delve into the possible reasons behind participants' involvement. We argue that intrinsic motivation — which is referred to an individual's willingness to engage in a behavior despite absence of any explicit reward arrangement (8) — could be a major reason. The students may participate in an activity to obtain feelings of accomplishment, satisfaction, or pleasure. In other words, the activity itself may constitute a reward so long as the prospective participants see the intrinsic values of the current program (e.g., the program being meaningful or itself constituting an avenue for personal growth). Thus, intrinsically motivated students may still partake in the program in spite of the absence of any explicit, tangible reward arrangements. In short, if an activity is inherently attractive or meaningful, individuals could be expected to engage in certain goal-directed behaviors with the objective to receive an internal reward. Internally motivated behaviors comprise interest, competence, curiosity, and self-actualization (9). These factors represent the key elements behind an individual's intrinsic motivation to participate in a program.

Clearly, a *good program design* is also instrumental to effective implementation of any programs. The demonstrated learning effect of students can be explained by the content of the program (10-11). A program whose content is compatible with the students' interests and abilities is bound to induce excitement and involvement from the participants. Program design comprises three elements, namely, activity-based learning, cooperative learning, and intensive training sessions. Hands-on experiments and activities form the basis of effective learning in activity-based learning. The concept of activity-based learning is rooted in the assertion that students are active learners rather than passive recipients of information. Excellent learning outcomes may be obtained by incorporating activities that warrants the active participation of students. Cooperative learning has been proven to improve the students' learning performances (12-17). Previous research revealed that group learning promotes mutual helping, interdependence among group members, interaction within the group, and interpersonal skills of individuals. Holding intensive training sessions in summer adds to the success of the program by ensuring the availability of student participants and offering them chances to meet one another.

Furthermore, *good professional skills and techniques* are indispensable for program success. Most program implementers had extensive experience in running the P.A.T.H.S. Project. The social workers identified 'group work skills' as a key to the effectiveness of the program. They observed positive changes in the students in both intrapersonal and interpersonal aspects. In the debriefing session, these social workers stated their observations and allowed them some time for self-reflection. Given their expertise on adolescent development, these social workers were able to facilitate the students' self-reflection and accordingly help the latter build a positive self-image. In addition, they endeavored to instill a culture of appreciation among the current student sample with a relatively low self-esteem. The compliments from social workers, teachers, and fellow group members are very powerful tools in building the self-esteem of students. These compliments, in conjunction with the self-recognition and the sense of accomplishment that students may derive along the program, would no doubt form the building block of self-esteem on which students could develop a positive mind-set.

Finally, the *involvement of teachers* significantly contributed to the success of the program. The school principal required the teachers to participate in the program, thereby motivating these teachers to facilitate the growth of their students. These teachers were also surprised by the strengths or hidden positive attributes of their students. For instance, those students who perform poorly in their studies might demonstrate excellent creativity and/or specific skills throughout the program. By looking at their students through a more holistic lens, teachers can provide their students with opportunities to develop themselves in different aspects. Furthermore, teachers may applaud their students for any improvement whereby such a positive feedback is massively rewarding to the latter. The social workers also alluded to the strong association between teacher's expressed appreciations and students' performance. Therefore, school teachers are considered helpful and crucial partners in the implementation of the project.

This research is not without its limitations. First, the lack of control groups at present does not permit us to rule out confounds such as maturation (18). Second, as a qualitative study, this paper cannot conveniently evaluate the impact of each factor which thus allows us to identify the most influential factor. We also cannot decipher the interweaving dynamics among various factors. Third, the fact that we only managed to locate two students for interviews may constitute a blow to the representativeness of the current sample. Despite these limitations, the findings suggest that the Project P.A.T.H.S. had positive impact on the student participants, while such an effect would hinge on several factors.

ACKNOWLEDGMENTS

The Project P.A.T.H.S. and the preparation for this paper were financially supported by The Hong Kong Jockey Club Charities Trust. This paper is based on an article published in the International Journal on Disability and Human Development 2018;17(3) issue. We thank the workers and students for joining this study.

APPENDIX A. GUIDE FOR INTERVIEW WITH SOCIAL WORKERS (PROCESS EVALUATION)

Tier 1 Program

1. Please briefly introduce the Tier 1 adolescent development program.
2. Which programs or activities would induce changes in adolescents? What kind of changes? What are the factors that lead to such changes (student factors, social worker intervention, collaborative relationship between social workers and students, program design, nature of programs, school administration assistance, and time and venue)?

Tier 2 Program

1. What criteria did you follow in recruiting the Tier 2 Program participants?
2. Please briefly introduce the Tier 2 adolescent development program.
3. Which programs or activities would induce changes in adolescents? What kind of changes? What are the factors that lead to such changes (student factors, social worker intervention, collaborative relationship between social workers and students, program design, nature of programs, school administration assistance, and time and venue)?

General comments about the program

1. In general, how would you evaluate the effectiveness of the Project P.A.T.H.S.?
2. What are the most successful aspects of the Project P.A.T.H.S.?

REFERENCES

[1] Branden N. The six pillars of self-esteem. Accessed 2016 Oct 25. URL:http://www.nathanielbranden.com/on-self-esteem
[2] Reasoner RW. Pro: You can bring hope to failing students. What's behind self-esteem programs: Truth or trickery? School Administrator 1992;49(4):23-4.
[3] Borba M, Taylor-McMillan B. Esteem builders: A K-8 self-esteem curriculum for improving student achievement, behavior, and school climate. Rolling Hills Estates, CA: Jalmar Press, 1989.
[4] Kolb DA. Experiential learning: Experience as the source of learning and development. Englewood Cliffs, NJ: Prentice-Hall, 1983.
[5] Shek DTL, Ma HK. Subjective outcome evaluation of the Project P.A.T.H.S.: Findings based on the perspective of the program participants. ScientificWorldJournal 2007;7:47-55.
[6] Shek DTL, Siu AMH, Lee TY. Subjective outcome evaluation of the Project P.A.T.H.S.: Findings based on the perspective of the program implementers. ScientificWorldJournal 2007;7:195-203.
[7] Shek DTL, Sun RCF. Subjective outcome evaluation of the Project P.A.T.H.S.: Qualitative findings based on the experiences of program implementers. ScientificWorldJournal 2007;7:1024-35.
[8] Shek DTL, Sun RCF. Subjective outcome evaluation of the Project P.A.T.H.S.: Qualitative findings based on the experiences of program participants. ScientificWorldJournal 2007;7:686-97.
[9] Deci EL. Intrinsic motivation. New York: Springer, 1975.
[10] Nicholls JG. Development of perception of own attainment and causal attributions for success and failure in reading. J Educ Psychol 1979;71(1):94-9.
[11] Anderson LW, Pellicer LO. Toward an understanding of unusually successful programs for economically disadvantaged students. J Educ Stud Placed Risk 1998;3(3):237-63.
[12] Yamarik S. Does cooperative learning improve student learning outcomes? J Econ Educ 2007;38(3):259-77.

[13] Ellis AK. Cooperative learning. In: Ellis AK, ed. Research on educational innovations. Larchmont, NY: Eye on Education, 2001:104-17.
[14] Rohrbeck CA, Ginsburg-Block MD, Fantuzzo JW, Miller TR. Peer-assisted learning interventions with elementary school students: A meta-analytic review. J Educ Psychol 2003;95(2):240-57.
[15] Slavin RE, Hurley EA, Chamberlain A. Cooperative learning and achievement: Theory and research. In: Reynolds WM, Miller GE, eds. Handbook of psychology. Hoboken, NJ: John Wiley, 2003:177-98.
[16] Slavin RE. Cooperative learning and intergroup relations. In: Banks J, ed. Handbook of research on multicultural education. New York: Macmillan, 1995:628-34.
[17] Slavin RE. Educational psychology: Theory and practice. New Jersey: Pearson, 2009.
[18] Campbell DT, Stanley JC. Experimental and quasi-experimental designs for research. Boston: Houghton Mifflin Company,1963.

In: Psychosocial Needs
Editors: Daniel TL Shek et al.

ISBN: 978-1-53611-951-0
© 2017 Nova Science Publishers, Inc.

Chapter 5

IDENTIFICATION OF SUCCESS FACTORS OF THE COMMUNITY-BASED ADOLESCENT PROJECT

Ben Law[1],*, PhD
and Daniel TL Shek[2-6], PhD, FHKPS, BBS, SBS, JP

[1]Department of Social Work and Social Administration, The University of Hong Kong, Hong Kong, PR China, [2]Department of Applied Social Sciences, The Hong Kong Polytechnic University, Hong Kong, PR China, [3]Centre for Innovative Programmes for Adolescents and Families, The Hong Kong Polytechnic University, Hong Kong, PR China, [4]Department of Social Work, East China Normal University, Shanghai, PR China, [5]Kiang Wu Nursing College of Macau, Macau, PR China and [6]Division of Adolescent Medicine, Department of Pediatrics, Kentucky Children's Hospital, University of Kentucky School of Medicine, Lexington, Kentucky, US

---

* Correspondence: Ben Law, PhD, Department of Social Work and Social Administration, The University of Hong Kong, Pokfulam Road, Hong Kong, PR China. Email: blaw@hku.hk.

In this chapter we try to identify the success factors in the community-based P.A.T.H.S. Project in Hong Kong. A qualitative study was conducted to collect views from social workers and program workers. Subjective evaluation reports filled by program participants and instructors were also used to support the findings of the focus group interviews. Results showed that the following factors contributed to positive program effects: 1) close relationship between instructors and participants; 2) good program design; 3) good professional skills and techniques of instructors; 4) smooth administrative management; and 5) presence of helping teachers. In conjunction with previous findings, the present study demonstrates the positive impact of the Tier 2 Program of the Project P.A.T.H.S. in promoting positive development of Chinese high school students in Hong Kong.

INTRODUCTION

Adolescence is a transitional period where numerous and stressful developmental tasks are involved (1–3). According to Erikson (1), adolescents face an identity crisis by resolving the conflict between ego identity and role confusion. The successful resolution of the conflict can develop the virtue of "fidelity". Newman and Newman (2), and Simpson and Roehlkepartain (3) further proposed specific types of developmental tasks in adolescence, such as advanced cognitive reasoning and responsibilities.

Apart from the general developmental approach, cultural perspective must also be considered to comprehensively conceptualize the development of Chinese adolescents in Hong Kong. The developmental issues for adolescents in Hong Kong are unique (4). One unique issue is the morbid emphasis on academic excellence, which was traditionally regarded as the ladder of social mobility. Therefore, adolescents in Hong Kong face serious academic stress, especially during public examinations. Most parents perceive that academic success is significantly more important than other aspects for an ideal child (5).

In order to help adolescents to develop in a holistic manner, the Positive Adolescent Training through Holistic Social Programs (the Project P.A.T.H.S)was initiated by The Hong Kong Jockey Club Charities Trust.

Based on the review of Catalano et al. (6) and considering the unique adolescent developmental issues in Hong Kong, a two-tier program with 15 positive youth development constructs was designed and implemented. The two tiers of the program are the Tier 1 Program and the Tier 2 Program. The Tier 1 Program is a 10- to 20-hour universal youth enhancement program for junior secondary school students (Secondary 1 to Secondary 3). Tier 2 Program is used to further cater to adolescents with high psychosocial needs.

The programs in the Initial Implementation Phase were implemented from 2005 to 2009. Considering the positive outcomes of the Project P.A.T.H.S., The Hong Kong Jockey Club Charities Trust further approved funding to implement an Extension Phase (2009-2016) and a three-year community-based project entitled "P.A.T.H.S. to Adulthood: A Jockey Club Community-Based Youth Enhancement Program" (community-based Project P.A.T.H.S. hereinafter) from January 2013 to August 2017 with two batches of applications (7-10). For the community-based project, the Tier 1 Program was more flexible. The service unit could use existing P.A.T.H.S. materials or develop additional units, provided that the target was a larger community.

This chapter documents the experience from the community-based Project P.A.T.H.S. conducted by the Tung Wah Group of Hospitals (TWGHs) in Hong Kong. The TWGHs has participated in the first batch of the program from January 2013 to December 2015. The corresponding service unit rendering the services is one of the Integrated Services Centre of TWGHs. The service unit launched the program at four secondary schools, ranging from schools admitting students with highest academic attainment (Band 1 schools) to schools admitting students with lowest academic attainment in the Central, Western, Southern, and Islands Districts.

A total of 638 students from four schools joined the Tier 1 Program rendered by TWGHs, and two modes were adopted for the schools in the program (i.e., Mode A for 2 schools and Mode B for 2 schools). Mode A program package focused on five positive youth development constructs, including behavioral competence (BC), moral competence (MC), self-efficacy (SE), clear and positive identity (ID), and prosocial norms (PN). In addition to exploring the interests and potential of students and enhancing their personal skills, the programs also aimed to foster the integration of adolescents and elderly in the community through service learning. There were three implementation stages for the service learning, including skills training, volunteer service, and debriefing. In the skills training stage, briefing of the program, training on communication skills, interviewing skills of narrative therapy, basic photography skills, and basic make-up techniques were introduced to the students before the service was delivered to the elderly. In the second implementation stage (volunteer service), the students, in a group of four to five, were required to interview one senior citizen. They had to collect information to create a personalized life story album for the senior citizens, and thus put their knowledge into practice. Students were encouraged to provide individual make-up and photography services for each elder participant. After the service delivery, a life story album and a photo frame made by the students were given to the elder interviewee as a gift. In the third stage of debriefing, students summarized their experiences after service delivery. An awarding ceremony was also held to celebrate the participation and effort of students in the program. Table 1 shows the service delivery process for Mode A.

The Mode B program package focused on personal growth education. For schools adopting the Mode B program package, school teachers were responsible for the implementation of the program. They were technically supported by social workers and program workers. The program mainly focused on several positive youth development constructs, including the promotion of behavioral competence (BC) and moral competence (MC), development of self-efficacy (SE), clear and positive identity (ID), and fostering prosocial norms (PN).

Regarding the Tier 2 Program, only two out of the four secondary schools participated because these two schools had more students with greater psychosocial needs. Given the selective nature of the Tier 2 Program, the students with relatively low self-esteem, weak social functioning, and poor academic results were the potential participants. The screening process for suitable participants was conducted by teachers and social workers by means of observation and interviews.

Table 1. Tier 1 Program plan for mode A

Tier 1 Program				
Preparation stage				
No. of Sessions	Theme	Content	Format	No. of participants
1	Briefing	- Introduction to narrative therapy	Workshop	All students
1	Elderly communication	- Learning how to communicate with the elderly	Talk Role play Training workshop	All students
1	Narrative therapy: interview skills training	- Learning interview skills of narrative therapy	Training workshop	All students
1	Basic photography skills	- Learning basic photography skills	Training workshop	All students
1	Basic make-up skills	- Learning basic make-up skills	Training workshop	All students
Service Delivery				
1	Service delivery	- Interview	Activity	All students
Debriefing Session				
1	Organizing data and creating booklets Evaluation	- Organizing data - Creating booklets for interviewees as gifts - Evaluation	Group	All students

As the Tier 2 Program for these two schools, a leadership training program called the Youth Volunteer Leadership Training Program was implemented. Leadership was used as the entry point for adolescents with greater psychosocial needs. As young people need nurturance and development, leadership training in the education sector has become increasingly important. *Leadership* denotes the ability of one member of a group to encourage other members to get things done, as well as maintain good relations within the group and organize group activities and ensure that they happen (11). Human development consists of two essential qualities, namely "excellence" and "ethics" (12). *Excellence* refers to intelligence and skills, while *ethics* refers to moral values and beliefs. Both qualities are important in leadership training. According to the needs of students in the local context, excellence is interpreted as "creativity" and "communications", while ethics is centered on "caring attitudes" and "commitment". Conducting a series of leadership training activities can possibly promote the excellence and ethics of all participants. In short, leadership is the process of building an individual's character strength and virtue.

By applying the concept of leadership suggested by Bennis and Nanus (13), everyone has the potential to become a leader. Each individual can demonstrate his or her leadership qualities under different contexts (13). The awareness of individuals on leadership within specific situational contexts is critical to developing this potential. Constant practice is the key to developing and maintaining the leadership qualities. Halloran and Benton (14) defined leadership simply as the ability to influence the action of others, in either formal or informal settings. Van and Fertman (15) defined three major stages of adolescent leadership development. The first stage is "awareness", in which the exploration of an individual's talents and potential for leadership is conducted with the assistance of others. The second stage is "growth and activity", in which teenagers gain a certain degree of confidence and leadership skills by participating in different kinds of activities. The third stage is "mastery", in which the mastery of specific skills is applied. Communication, decision-making, and stress management are cultivated when teenagers go through the three stages. Adolescents who complete one stage will go to the next stage to further develop their leadership qualities. However, if they encounter a new situation, they will go back to the previous stage. The Center for Creative Leadership, a USA research and training institute for leadership, demonstrated that leadership training consists of "challenging experience", "evaluation and reflection", and "encouragement". Challenge is a developmental force because it creates a condition where a leader must grow to be effective. When facing a new environment, relationship, and other things, leaders are forced to move from their comfort zones and to learn and grow.

Based on the above conceptual considerations, problem solving and adventure-based activities were designed in the Project P.A.T.H.S. for allowing participants to move beyond their comfort zones. For example, participants were given the task of planning a charitable event. Before leadership training, participants had to review their present level of leadership and estimate the discrepancy between their desired level and present level. They were encouraged to evaluate their achievement first after each challenging experience and then establish concrete goals and ways to improve. Reflection could enable participants to express their feelings and thoughts in the challenging experience. Instructors needed to give feedback and debrief the participants after each activity. Reflection and debriefing at the end of the program were performed to help the participants consolidate their learning. Participants moving from their comfort zones can have difficulty developing and growing without positive feedback and encouragement from others. Participants may end up failing and experiencing setbacks without such support. Hence, encouragement does not only boost their confidence but also creates a scenario where they can learn resilience. Instructors, teachers, parents, peers, and professionals are the best people to extend encouragements and compliments to participants. Encouraging participants can further strengthen their caring attitude.

According to Erikson, one must successfully resolve a crisis at each of the eight psychosocial stages of development to achieve a healthy personality (16). At the fifth stage (ego identity versus role confusion), teenagers have to examine their identities and the roles they occupy. They must achieve an integrated sense of self and identify what they want to do and be. If they fail to achieve these things, they will suffer from confusion about their different roles in the society, such as occupational, sexual, and religious roles. Adolescents usually experience identity crisis. The results of prolonged identity crisis are deviant behaviors, negative self-concept, and confusion towards the future. Participants in the Project P.A.T.H.S were expected to develop their identity by joining a series of experiential activities to cultivate leadership qualities, such as courage, communication, caring, and commitment.

The Tier 2 Program was conducted once in a year in each school. Two sessions were implemented for the briefing of the program and the recruitment of participants. After the opening sessions, six sessions of leadership training and group leading skills training were introduced to strengthen the self-esteem, character strength, and virtue as leaders of students. Then, volunteer service was designed and carried out in six sessions for students with the support of the program staff members and school teachers. After the completion of these tasks, one session for evaluation and review of the previous sessions, and the celebration of the program completion was held. Based on the performance and degree of participation of students, different awards, such as the Excellent Performance Award and the Best Improved Student Award, were given to students. In addition, a certificate of participation was given to students who achieved an attendance of 80% or above to increase the incentive of the students in attending the program sessions. At the end of the program, a graduation ceremony was held to celebrate their participation in the program, with the school principal, teachers, and parents as guests.

Among the various Tier 2 programs in the period from 2013 to 2015, two significant events were suggested by the program implementers to illustrate the effectiveness of the Tier 2 Program of P.A.T.H.S. conducted by the TWGHs' Jockey Club Lei Tung Integrated Services Centre. The objectives of the present study were to 1) collect data regarding evaluations on the post-event effect to the participating adolescents and social workers, 2) evaluate the positive effects of community-based Project P.A.T.H.S. on its service users, and 3) explore the factors that contribute to the positive youth development of junior secondary school students in Hong Kong.

OUR STUDY

Four schools joined the three-year community-based Project P.A.T.H.S conducted by an Integrated Services Centre of TWGHs in the school year 2013 to 2015. All four schools adopted the 10-hour Core Tier 1 Program while only two schools joined the Tier 2 Program. In the evaluation process, a focus group interview was held to collect opinions from program implementers (social workers and program workers) about the factors contributing to the success of the P.A.T.H.S Project. Meanwhile, researchers collected feedback from program implementers and student participants respectively, based on the Subjective Evaluation Reports after the completion of the Tier 2 program. Concerning the focus group interview, program implementers, who were the informants, were notified of the purpose and confidentiality of the interview and were asked to sign the consent forms before the interview began. A trained research assistant with a master's degree in Social Work conducted the interview. The interview lasted for 50 minutes and was conducted in June 2016. The focus group interview was audio taped after obtaining consent from the informants. During the interview, the program implementers responsible for the programs were encouraged to verbalize their practice wisdom that they used to design and implement the program in different schools. The research assistant conducting the interview had training in social group work.

Regarding the evaluation based on consolidated reports, the consolidated data were integrated to form an overall profile. Participants and program implementers responded to Subjective Outcome Evaluation Forms (Forms A and B for the Tier 1 Program, and Forms C and D for the Tier 2 Program) to give their views after program completion (7–10). The consolidated data provide additional support to the findings from the focus group interview.

Instruments

The interview guide was specific, self-constructed, and semi-structured (Appendix A). The guide was divided into three parts:

Table 2. Number of schools, participants and program implementers participated in Tier 2 Program over three years

	2013	2014	2015
Number of school	2	2	2
Total number of core participants	80	80	80
S1	32	40	40
S2	40	40	40
S3	8	/	/
Program implementers	15	11	9

Table 3. General Tier 2 program

Name of Program: Youth Volunteer Leadership Training Program	
Goal of the project	The leadership qualities of all participants were expected to be promoted through a series of leadership training activities.
Specific aims	<ul><li>To strengthen the communication skills of participants</li><li>To enhance the courage of participants</li><li>To increase the sense of commitment of participants</li><li>To cultivate the caring attitude of participants towards others and the community</li></ul>
Covered constructs	<ul><li>Cultivation of resilience</li><li>Promotion of behavioral competence</li><li>Development of self-efficacy</li><li>Development of clear and positive identity</li><li>Recognition of positive behavior</li></ul>
General program plan	
Part one: Self-exploration	

No. of Sessions	Theme	Content	Format	No. of participants
2	Self-understanding	-Exploration of strengths and self-recognition	Group	80

Part two: Leadership Training Workshop/Camp

No. of Sessions	Theme	Content	Format	No. of participants
4	Leadership training (courage, communication, caring and commitment)	-Group discussion -Skill practice -Adventure	Workshop Training camp	80

Part three: Activity planning				
No. of sessions	Theme	Content	Format	No. of participants
5	Meeting and preparation before the implementation of the charitable event	-Planning a charitable event	Group	80
2	Charitable event	-Service delivery	Activity	80
Part four: Evaluation				
No. of sessions	Theme	Content	Format	No. of participants
2	Conclusion evaluation	-Sharing of feelings and thoughts of joining the program	Sharing session/ Ceremony	80

- Informants' views on the Tier 1 Program, such as the observed change in students and the major activities and factors contributing to the change in the students.
- Informants' views on the Tier 2 Program, such as the observed change in students and the major activities and factors contributing to the change in the students.
- Informants' general perceptions of the program's effectiveness and success.

The content of the tape-recorded interview was fully transcribed and checked for accuracy by a research assistant.

WHAT WE FOUND

For the Tier 1 Program, Mode B program was adopted in School A (Band 2) and School B (Band 3). School C and School D (both were Band 1 schools) adopted Mode A program.

Table 4. Significant events for the Tier 2 program in school A

Part A: Experiential activity — Reality Room Escape Game

• Goals
    • To enhance group cohesion of students
    • To equip students with resilience and decision-making ability
    • To increase the problem-solving skills of students

• Content
    • Beginner version of Reality Room Escape was set for students.
    • Reality Room Escape is a reality adventure game, in which players are locked in a room and have to use elements in the room to solve a series of puzzles and escape within a set time limit.
    • Games are set in a variety of fictional locations, such as maze, magic classrooms, and the principal's room, and are popular as team building exercises.

Part B: Workshop —Reality Room Escape Planning

• Goals
    • To learn the division of labor and cooperation
    • To learn effective interpersonal communication skills
    • To utilize imagination and creativity

• Content
    • Students formed several small groups and discussed the matter.
    • They were given a task of designing a reality escape game for other students.
    • In the process, they needed to assign individual roles and prepare materials.
    • Given their experience of playing the game and their creativity in designing the game, they were appointed as planners of the game.

Part C: Reality Room Escape Implementation

• Goals
    • To create a successful experience for student designers
    • To increase problem-solving skills of the student participants

• Content   • Put the game design into practice

Meanwhile, School A and School B were invited to participate in the Tier 2 Program, in which 80 Secondary 1 to Secondary 3 students participated in a 15-week program (excepted one which had one extra session) (Table 2). Social workers and program workers provided students with training for leadership, activity planning and implementation skills (Table 3). Students in School A were asked to develop a Room Escape Game at school; students in School B planned a school event to raise the awareness of school members towards the worldwide food wastage issue, and designed activities for Food Wise Day (refer to Table 4 and Table 5 for details of two events). These challenges were designed to train students' teamwork, problem-solving, communication and cooperation skills. Meanwhile, students could make friends with each other during the program. Over the three-year period, the Tier 2 Programs has been organized in the two schools for six and seven times respectively.

The focus group interviews with program implementers and the consolidated data from the subjective evaluation from participants and program implementers provided evidence on the positive effect of the community-based Project P.A.T.H.S. for the participants. Consolidating the feedback from the evaluation forms, many participants were satisfied with and had more positive than negative comments towards the program. Participants rated on the program implementation, quality of program workers, and effectiveness of the program in the evaluation form (see Table 6). Over 90% of the participants from various Tier 2 programs were satisfied with how the program was designed and organized by the workers, and acknowledged that the program was effective in their personal development. From their written feedback, participants appreciated the smooth implementation of the program, and they found that activities were challenging, fruitful and meaningful. Participants especially treasured the opportunities to have outdoor and adventure-based activities. Concerning their views towards the program implementers, participant generally found the implementers were well-prepared, friendly and thoughtful, and would actively care about their needs with a warm attitude. Most importantly, participants found the program to be beneficial to their personal growth. They perceived that the program promoted adolescent development, including interpersonal skills, caring attitude for others and community, problem-solving skills, resilience, team work, and confidence.

Table 5. Significant events for the Tier 2 program in school B

Theme: Global Hunger — Who Rules The World?
Part A: Workshop — Global Hunger

• Goals
    • To increase the understanding of students on global hunger issue
    • To raise the awareness of students on the importance of food

• Content
    • Poverty issues in Hong Kong
    • Global hunger
    • Global food culture

Part B: Workshop — Food Ambassador Training

• Goals
    • To learn the division of labor and cooperation
    • To learn effective interpersonal communication skills
    • To raise awareness of students on the importance of food

• Content
    • Students formed several small groups and discussed the matter.
    • They were given a task of designing activities for "Food Wise Day", which was a day to promote the message of food appreciation.
    • In the process, they needed to assign individual roles and prepare materials.

Part C: Food Wise Day

• Goals
    • To increase the understanding of students on global hunger issue
    • To raise awareness of students on the importance of food
    • To create a successful experience for student designers

• Content
    • Food ambassadors were responsible for the implementation of Food Wise Day.
    • Student participants were divided into two groups: the rich and poor groups. Only a small portion of student participants were in the rich group while the majority of them were in the poor group. They were encouraged to experience the lunch of two groups and reflect on the issue of global hunger and the importance of food.

Meanwhile, the program implementers found that the program were well prepared and delivered, which also had a great positive influence on the development of the participants (see table 7). They understood more about the thoughts and needs of adolescents. Some also pointed out the importance of experiential learning for inspiring and motivating participants.

Table 6. Feedback from participants collected from evaluation forms

	2013		2014		2015		Overall	
	Mean	SD	Mean	SD	Mean	SD	Mean	SD
Views towards the program								
S1	4.82	.79	4.82	.84	5.05	.64	4.90	.76
S2	5.40	.61	5.09	.60	5.02	.34	5.17	.55
S3	4.95	.77	N/A	N/A	N/A	N/A	4.95	.77
Overall	5.12	.75	4.96	.74	5.03	.51	5.04	.68
Views towards the workers								
S1	4.82	.79	4.82	.84	5.05	.64	4.90	.76
S2	5.40	.61	5.09	.60	5.02	.34	5.17	.55
S3	4.95	.77	N/A	N/A	N/A	N/A	4.95	.77
Overall	5.12	.75	4.96	.74	5.03	.51	5.04	.68
Perceived effectiveness of the program	4.82	.79	4.82	.84	5.05	.64	4.90	.76
S1	5.40	.61	5.09	.60	5.02	.34	5.17	.55
S2	4.95	.77	N/A	N/A	N/A	N/A	4.95	.77
S3	5.12	.75	4.96	.74	5.03	.51	5.04	.68
Overall	4.82	.79	4.82	.84	5.05	.64	4.90	.76
	5.40	.61	5.09	.60	5.02	.34	5.17	.55

Note: Participants rated from 1 (strongly disagree) to 6 (strongly agree).

Concluding from the Tier 2 Program, the program implementers observed gradual improvement among participants. They agreed that the program promoted the participants' creativity and decision-making skills. Participants were observed to have a clearer sense of identity, and were more capable of caring about others and shouldering responsibilities. Program implementers generally concluded that the Tier 2 Program had positive impacts on participants' personal growth and interpersonal relationship.

Table 7. Feedback from program implementers collected from evaluation forms

	2013 N	2013 Mean	2013 SD	2014 N	2014 Mean	2014 SD	2015 N	2015 Mean	2015 SD	Overall N	Overall Mean	Overall SD
Views towards the program												
S1	6	5.06	.77	6	5.02	.87	4	4.91	.76	16	5.01	.75
S2	6	5.13	.70	5	5.18	.59	5	4.88	.20	16	5.06	.53
S3	3	.46	.54	N/A	N/A	N/A	N/A	N/A	N/A	3	.46	.54
Overall	15	5.00	.68	11	5.09	.72	9	4.89	.49	35	5.00	.64
Views towards the workers												
S1	6	5.13	.92	6	5.06	.84	4	5.41	.73	16	5.17	.80
S2	6	5.40	.54	5	5.13	.61	5	5.15	.16	16	5.23	.47
S3	3	4.83	.76	N/A	N/A	N/A	N/A	N/A	N/A	3	4.83	.76
Overall	15	5.18	.73	11	5.09	.71	9	5.26	.48	35	5.17	.65
Perceived effectiveness of the program												
S1	6	5.13	.92	6	4.77	.96	4	4.56	.41	16	4.85	.82
S2	6	5.00	.86	5	5.03	.69	5	4.95	.33	16	4.99	.63
S3	3	4.38	.54	N/A	N/A	N/A	N/A	N/A	N/A	3	4.38	.54
Overall	15	4.93	.83	11	4.89	.81	9	4.78	.40	35	4.88	.72

Note: Participants rated from 1 (strongly disagree) to 6 (strongly agree).

During the focus group interview, the program implementers quoted observations from teachers and school social workers. The students who participated in the program showed significant improvement in different aspects, such as their degree of participation, willingness to help others, earnestness when answering questions, and initiative and cooperative behaviors. The program implementers expressed that they were satisfied with the improvement and performance in the program participants.

The findings of focus group interviews and the consolidated reports showed that several factors contributed to the development of junior secondary school students. They are presented in the following paragraphs.

Good relationship between program implementers and students

The focus group interviews indicated that relationship building was perceived by program implementers as the most important and fundamental step in the program. They adopted an "egalitarian" position in which the participants and program implementers were involved. Power was seldom used by the program implementers unless mutual respect was violated because of the inappropriate behavior of participants. The implementers emphasized that they were not teachers giving lessons, but they sincerely hoped that the participants would try their best to provide constructive feedback. Based on observations by the teachers and instructors, students gave more responses in class discussion, answered questions seriously, and accepted the instructors. The "egalitarian" position received positive feedback from program participants. According to the Subjective Evaluation Reports responded by participants, most of the comments given to program implementers were regarding their good and friendly attitude.

Good program design

Several aspects of the program design contributed to its effectiveness. First, the latest video clips and newspaper articles were used instead of the original P.A.T.H.S. materials. To attract the attention of students in the Tier 1 Program, instructors had to find significantly interesting and up-to-date materials to deliver their message. During the focus group interview, the respondents mentioned that "students will not fall sleep easily if the video or news article is up to date," and "some current episodes of TV programs are interesting and attract the attention of students." Second, several in-class activities, group discussion, and reflection questions were also introduced to draw the attention of the students. The interactive mode adopted in the Tier 1 Program can help keep the students in the program.

Third, adjustments were conducted, such as incorporating additional activities that involve talking rather than writing for students who came from lower banding schools or those with special educational needs. Fourth, multiple sessions instead of a single session were adopted to ensure better learning for students. For example, a few workshops and experiential activities were conducted before the implementation of the "Reality Escape Game" and the "Food Wise Day". The step-by-step learning enhanced the effect of the program. Finally, the interest of students was considered in the program implementation. The program implementers mentioned that the degree of student participation increases with their interest in the program. For example, students were motivated to join the program when they participated in the Reality Escape Game. This hands-on experience is a driving force for them to design a school version of the Reality Escape Game for their schoolmates.

Good skills and techniques of program implementers

Apart from relationship building and designing of the program, the skills and techniques used by the program implementers also contributed to the success of the program. Their rich work experiences with the youth provided the program implementers (interviewees in the focus group) with numerous skills and techniques that could be employed in the intervention. Regarding the role of program implementers, the position of a facilitator was emphasized by the interviewees in the focus group. One interviewee said that "my job is to provide assistance when necessary, such as giving them (students) directions and helping them in brainstorming." In the interview, one of the interviewees mentioned that "the students are in charge of the events (Reality Escape Game and Food Wise Day)." This response implied that the program implementers emphasized the students' ownership, responsibility, and decision making in the event. Another interviewee stated that "my role is to remind them about the practicality of the proposed activities. I told them that their functions would influence the entire event and they (students) therefore should do their best to make the event a successful one." Second, the program implementers also employed contracting. Contracting is a practical skill used to set up the contract with the participants. Two main rules were set by the program implementers: mutual respect and active participation. One interviewee mentioned that "we are not teachers. We allow talking in class (the Tier 1 Program) but the voice should not be too loud and disturbing." Active participation is the key to a successful program. Hence, program implementers encouraged the participants to feel free in giving responses in class.

Third, prizes and praises were given to encourage participants to provide additional responses. One interviewee said that "snacks and sweets are very desirable to students. They answer questions whenever snacks and sweets are given." Apart from the tangible reward, verbal compliment is also a powerful tool to increase the participation of students. Fourth, program implementers intervened in conflict resolution. One interviewee stated that "when they (students) are in conflict, we (program implementers) calm them down and allow them to think of the pros and cons of their decision, educate them to think from different perspectives and understand others, and emphasize the importance of listening." Finally, briefing and debriefing techniques were emphasized by the interviewees and were used at the start and end of a session. For example, a discussion on global hunger, distribution of resources, fairness, equality, and poverty in Hong Kong (briefing) were conducted before the introduction of "Food Wise Day". After the end of each session, the program implementers helped the participants evaluate their performance and the progress of their preparation for the activity (debriefing).

Good administrative arrangement

The focus group interviewees mentioned that good administrative arrangement played a significant role in the success of the program. The administrative arrangement included shared workload among teachers, organized lesson schedules, briefing with teachers before program implementation, and collaboration between different parties. Before the implementation of the program, the program coordinator usually introduced the project to the staff, including the year's main theme, goals of the project, and program plan. The school could then conduct an early preparation because of the early notification to the teachers who are responsible for teaching the Tier 1 Program. In the community-based Project P.A.T.H.S, lesson schedules were arranged efficiently, especially for the Tier 1 Program, because of the support from school principals and relevant teachers. In addition, teachers acting as program implementers in the Tier 1 Program expanded the manpower of the program. Class teachers who knew their students well were selected to be helpers in the Tier 1 Program. The existing relationship between teachers and students made the teachers' roles essential in teaching the Tier 1 Program. Social workers stationed in the schools liaised with social workers and program workers from the Integrated Youth Service Team in the district to support the project. Therefore, collaboration among teachers, social workers, and program workers contributed to the good administrative management of the project. The results from the Forms B and D of the Subjective Evaluation Report demonstrated that the collaboration among the program implementers was excellent.

Helpful teachers

The role of teachers was essential for the success of the community-based P.A.T.H.S. Project. Some teachers were responsible for teaching the Tier 1 Program. They were capable of teaching the program because of their past experiences of conducting the school-based P.A.T.H.S. programs. The teachers were familiar with the aims, content, as well as the possible difficulties and solutions of the program. In addition to the teachers who were responsible for the Tier 1 Program, class teachers also played an important role in assisting program implementers, particularly the social workers and program workers from the Integrated Youth Service Team. Class teachers provided classroom management, including the supervision of the inappropriate behaviors and disciplinary problems of students, to ensure that the sessions of the Tier 1 Program were well organized. One interviewee mentioned that "teachers would remind students to be careful and not to display any inappropriate behavior. This approach helped me significantly." Moreover, they also provided program implementers with some basic information about the class, such as who among the students needed extra attention and would possibly display behavioral or emotional problems. With the early notification from class teachers, the program implementers better prepared for the program sessions.

Limitations of Tier 2 program

In spite of the five contributing factors that the program implementers had suggested in the focus group interview, there were some comments in the evaluation forms stating the limitations of the Tier 2 program, which might discount program effectiveness. For instance, there were limited number and length of sessions, instead of a long-term developmental program, for the implementers to coach and establish trusting relationships with the participants. Additionally, working in school settings, program implementers needed to consider the manpower and resources of the school, and as well as the school schedule. Such contextual restrictions might restrict the program implementers from organizing various innovative activities for participants and maximizing the benefits of the program.

DISCUSSION

The primary objective of this study was to identify factors that contributed to the success in the community-based P.A.T.H.S. Project. The study showed that several factors contributed to a successful community-based positive youth development program. The accounts of the interviewees and consolidated data clearly indicated that the close relationship between instructors and participants, good program design, good professional skills and techniques of instructors, good administrative management, and helpful role of teachers were the major factors that contributed to the successful implementation of the community-based P.A.T.H.S. Project. These findings are consistent with previous research on successful P.A.T.H.S. programs. Specifically, Shek and Sun (17) suggested that the 5 "P" factors, including policy, people, program, process and place, were highly contributing to the successful implementation of youth developmental programs.

Primarily, the present findings suggest that close relationship between instructors and participants is important. Traditionally, the relationship between service users and social workers is "the heart of social work" (18). As reported in the focus group interview, the program implementers' strong mindset of relationship building ensured the close relationship between the instructors and participants. A caring and supportive attitude is one of the important factors that promote youth leadership and intrapersonal development (19). Some comments were as follows: "instructors are considerate, friendly, caring, and willing to interact with them." The findings of the subjective evaluation also showed that students enjoyed their time with program implementers, because they were respected, valued, and supported in the program.

The present findings also suggest that good program design is important. In fact, a good program design is crucial to the outcome of any program. The demonstrated learning effect of students can be explained by the content of the program (20). If the content of the program is suitable for students in terms of their interests and abilities, then students can enjoy the excitement from joining the program and are willing to accept challenges in the program. On the basis of the findings from research, the following five elements of good program design were found: 1) good preparation of up-to-date materials; 2) interactive program; 3) reasonable adjustment based on the needs of schools; 4) the use of multiple sessions; and 5) focus on the interests of students.

Good professional skills and techniques of the instructors are also of paramount importance to program success. In this study, most instructors had rich working experiences of conducting the Tier 1 Program. The focus group interviewees acknowledged that their youth work experience and the teachers' skills in handling the Tier 1 Program contributed to the effectiveness of the program. Before implementation, most of the instructors received sufficient training provided by the Integrated Services Centre. They were equipped with specific knowledge and skills on how to implement the program. According to the Subjective Evaluation Report filled by students and instructors, instructors were perceived as competent and well prepared. For social workers in charge of the Tier 2 Program, their social work training further contributed to the success of the program. Briefing and debriefing skills, conflict resolution skills, contracting techniques, and behavioral modification techniques were adopted by the program workers, as reported in the focus group interview.

Good administrative support is also vital to successful program implementation. Administratively, the school needed to fit the program into the school policy and provide administrative support for the program implementers. Research showed that with strong support and leadership of school principals, the Project P.A.T.H.S. can be implemented successfully (21-24). The principal's level of commitment to the program, organizational skills, and ability to motivate staff members contributed to the coherence and implementation of the program (25). Positive attitudes of administrators and teachers can further improve the implementation of the program (22). Based on the present findings, the factors that helped facilitate program execution of the community-based Project P.A.T.H.S are as follows: 1) briefing session arranged before implementation; 2) sufficient time for early preparation; 3) making lessons to be a part of the school curriculum; 4) shared workload among teachers; 5) the use of good manpower deployment strategies to form a supportive team, and 6) collaboration among different involved parties.

Finally, teachers play a significant role in the successful implementation of the programs of the P.A.T.H.S. Project. Specifically, responsible and self-motivated teachers are important facilitating factors in the program. The roles of the teachers, instructors, and helpers contributed significantly to the success of the community-based P.A.T.H.S. programs. Their abundant experience in teaching the Tier 1 Program helped maximize the learning of the students. With the support from class teachers, program implementers can adjust their intervention styles on the basis of the information given by class teachers. The present findings further reinforced the importance of helpful teachers when implementing the P.A.T.H.S. programs.

The findings from present studies echo part of the 5 "P"s framework proposed by Shek and Sun (18). It re-states the importance of an interactive program with developmentally appropriate content (Program), as it could increase the motivation of adolescents to participate in and gain positive outcomes from the program. Moreover, social workers, program workers and teachers worked closely together to manage the class as well as to ensure a warm and respecting atmosphere (People). This could encourage participants to participate in the activities, and build up close relationships with implementers and other students. Meanwhile, from the suggestions of program implementers, having a better coordination with school and a suitable environment to implement the program (Policies and Place) could help maximize the effectiveness of the program. Overall, the whole process, including the preparation and design of program, program implementation, and participations of implementers and students were all vital elements for a successful youth developmental program (Process).

Several limitations of this study must be highlighted. First, as many factors may possibly contribute to an effective positive youth development program, the study may have missed some factors, such as the readiness of the students to engage in the programs. Second, the present study cannot give the degree of importance of each factor or demonstrate the complex relationship among the factors. However, the present study can account for the effectiveness of the program and encourage further studies on the factors contributing to an effective positive youth development program. Third, social desirability may result from the self-reported evaluation. Workers may have a self-fulfilling prophecy that they maintained the view that the programs worked well. Fourth, since the present study only covered the views of the implementers, further studies involving the students would be helpful. The research team compensated for the limitation of this study to some extent by using consolidated data as supportive evidence. Despite these limitations, the present findings suggested that the community-based Project P.A.T.H.S. had a positive effect on the participating students and possible factors were suggested to account for the effectiveness of the program.

ACKNOWLEDGMENTS

The Project P.A.T.H.S. and the present paper were financially supported by The Hong Kong Jockey Club Charities Trust. This paper is based on an article published in the International Journal on Disability and Human Development 2018;17(3) issue. We thank the workers and participants for joining this study.

Appendix A. Guide for interview with responsible program staff members (Process evaluation)

Tier 1 Program

1. Please briefly introduce the Tier 1 Program for adolescent development.
2. Which programs or activities would bring significant changes to adolescents? What were these changes? What factors (student factors, social worker intervention, collaborative relationship between social workers and students, program design, nature of programs, school administration assistance, and time and venue) would lead to change?

Tier 2 Program

1. What were the criteria in recruiting the Tier 2 Program participants?
2. Please briefly introduce the Tier 2 Program for adolescent development.
3. Which programs or activities would bring significant changes to adolescents? What were these changes? What factors (student factors, social worker intervention, collaborative relationship between social workers and students, program design, nature of programs, school administration assistance, and time and venue) would lead to change?

General comments to the program

1. How would you evaluate the overall effectiveness of the community-based Project P.A.T.H.S.?
2. In your own view, what aspects of the community-based Project P.A.T.H.S. were successful?

REFERENCES

[1] Erikson EH. Childhood and society, revised edition. New York: Norton, 1963.
[2] Newman BM, Newman PR. Development through life: A psychosocial approach. Homewood, IL: Dorsey Press, 1984.
[3] Simpson AR, Roehlkepartain JL. Asset building in parenting practices and family life. In: Lerner RM, Benson PL, eds. Developmental assets and asset-building communities: Implications for research, policy and practice. New York: Kluwer Academic Plenum, 2003:157–93.
[4] Shek DTL. Social stress in Hong Kong. In: Estes J, ed. Social development index. Hong Kong: Oxford University Press, 2005:213-22.
[5] Shek DTL, Chan LK. Hong Kong Chinese parents' perceptions of the ideal child. J Psychol 1999;133(3):291-302.
[6] Catalano RF, Berglund ML, Ryan JAM, Lonczak HS, Hawkins JD. Positive youth development in the United States: Research findings on evaluations of positive youth development programs. Ann Am Acad Polit SS 2004;591(1):98–124.
[7] Shek DTL, Ma HK. Subjective outcome evaluation of the Project P.A.T.H.S.: Findings based on the perspective of the program participants. ScientificWorldJournal 2007;7:47-55.
[8] Shek DTL, Siu AMH, Lee TY. Subjective outcome evaluation of the Project P.A.T.H.S.: Findings based on the perspective of the program implementers. ScientificWorldJournal 2007;7:195-203.
[9] Shek DTL, Sun RCF. Subjective outcome evaluation of the Project P.A.T.H.S.: Qualitative findings based on the experiences of the program implementers. ScientificWorldJournal 2007;7:1024-35.
[10] Shek DTL, Sun RCF. Subjective outcome evaluation of the Project P.A.T.H.S.: Qualitative findings based on the experiences of the program participants. ScientificWorldJournal 2007;7:686-97.
[11] Peterson C, Seligman MEP. Character strengths and virtues: A handbook and classification. New York: Oxford University Press and Washington, DC: American Psychological Association, 2004.
[12] Gardner H, Csikszentmihalyi M, Damon W. Good work: When excellence and ethics meet. New York: Basic Books, 2001.
[13] Bennis WG, Nanus B. Leaders: The strategies for taking charge. New York: Harper & Row, 1985.
[14] Halloran J, Benton D. Applied human relations: An organizational approach. Englewood Cliffs, NJ: Prentice Hall, 1987.
[15] Van Linden JA, Fertman CI. Youth leadership: A guide to understanding leadership development in adolescents. San Francisco, CA: Jossey-Bass, 1998.
[16] Erikson EH. Identity and life cycle. New York: W.W.Norton, 1959-1994.

[17] Shek DTL, Sun RCF. Implementation quality of a positive youth development program: Cross-case analyses based on seven cases in Hong Kong. ScientificWorldJournal 2008;8:1075-87.
[18] Collins J, Collins M. Achieving change in social work. London: Heinemann, 1981.
[19] Shek DTL, Wu FKY. The role of teachers in youth development: Reflections of students. Int J Disabil Human Dev 2014;13(4):473-80.
[20] Anderson LW, Pellicer LO. Toward an understanding of unusually successful programs for economically disadvantaged students. JESPAR 1998;3(3):237-63.
[21] Van Dalen J, Van Hout JCHM, Wolfhagen HAP, Scherpbier AJJA, Van Der Vleuten CPM. Factors influencing the effectiveness of communication skills training: Programme contents outweigh teachers' skills. Med Teach 1999;21(3):308-10.
[22] Frazee BM. Hawthorne elementary school: The university perspective. JESPAR 1996;1(1):25-31.
[23] George CA.; Grissom JB, Stories of mixed success: Program improvement implementation in Chapter 1 Schools. JESPAR 1996;1(1):77-93.
[24] Edmonds R. Effective schools for the urban poor. Educ Leadership 1979;37(1):15-24.
[25] Stringfield S. Attempting to enhance students' learning through Innovative Programs: The case for schools evolving into high reliability organizations. Sch Eff Sch Improv 1995;6 (1):67-96.

In: Psychosocial Needs
Editors: Daniel TL Shek et al.

ISBN: 978-1-53611-951-0
© 2017 Nova Science Publishers, Inc.

Chapter 6

FACTORS CONTRIBUTING TO THE SUCCESS IN LIFE AND CAREER

Janet TY Leung[1,], PhD and Daniel TL Shek[1-5], PhD, FHKPS, BBS, SBS, JP*

[1]Department of Applied Social Sciences,
The Hong Kong Polytechnic University, Hong Kong, PR China
[2]Centre for Innovative Programmes for Adolescents and Families,
The Hong Kong Polytechnic University, Hong Kong, PR China
[3]Department of Social Work, East China Normal University,
Shanghai, PR China
[4]Kiang Wu Nursing College of Macau, Macau, PR China
[5]Division of Adolescent Medicine, Department of Pediatrics,
Kentucky Children's Hospital,
University of Kentucky College of Medicine,
Lexington, Kentucky, US

---

[*] Correspondence: Janet Leung, PhD, Department of Applied Social Sciences, The Hong Kong Polytechnic University, Hunghom, Hong Kong, PR China. E-mail: janet.leung@polyu.edu.hk.

Based on the qualitative data collected from a case interview with the chief program implementer as well as focus group interviews with 57 Secondary 3 students in Hong Kong, factors contributing to the success of a life and career planning program adopting a positive youth development approach in a secondary school were examined. Six themes conducive to program success were extracted from the narratives: a) clear objectives with strong emphasis on adolescent psychosocial development, b) diverse and creative program design, c) experiential approach that allowed participants to experience, reflect and learn, d) quality implementers, e) continuous feedback from the participants, and f) good timing in launching the program. The factors suggest that the positive youth development approach provides a holistic framework of the design and content of the life and career development. Theoretical and practical implications of the study are discussed.

INTRODUCTION

Adolescents are the backbone of the future society. They search for self-identity and independence and develop their competencies so as to become independent, competent and responsible adults who make necessary contributions to the family, community and society. However, adolescents today might be too well-protected and better-nurtured by their parents. Generation theorists use different terminologies to describe the adolescents nowadays as Generation ME (1), the Net Generation (2), and the Millennials (3). The Millennials are portrayed as confident, sheltered and achieving individuals (3). But at the same time, the Generation ME are described as egocentric and narcissistic (1). Schneider and Stevenson (4) suggested that the youth today are motivated but directionless.

Life and career development has become a hot topic in the local and global contexts. According to the American Counseling Association, career development is the "total constellation of psychological, sociological, educational, physical, economic, and chance factors that combine to influence the nature and significance of work in the total life span of any given individual" (5, p.2). Under this definition, career development is the development of one's purposes, tasks and choices for the fulfillment of one's needs and life goals at different stages of life.

While some life and career development programs focus on personality-career match and vocational preparation (6,7), there are some programs that emphasize the personal development of the individuals (8,9). For instance, Solberg et al. (8) expanded the school-to-work (STW) intervention model to school-to-work-to-life (STWL) intervention model and paid more emphasis on helping the youth to develop their competencies so that they could adapt successfully to the changing environment. Sue et al. (9) developed a model of resilience that portrays how one's strengths and potential maximize one's mental health and emphasized the importance of middle school students to build up resiliency against adversity. These models echo the conceptual framework of positive youth development that emphasizes the assets, abilities and potential of adolescents (10, 11).

In Hong Kong, life planning education plays an overarching role in "fostering students' self-understanding, personal planning, goal setting, reflective habits of mind and articulation to progression pathways" (12, p.3). There are three components of life and career development: self-understanding and development, career exploration, and career planning and management. It has been emphasized that life and career development should be in line with the whole-person development and life-long learning (12). Unfortunately, life and career development in Hong Kong has been criticized as fragmented and superficial, with a narrow focus of information dissemination of educational and vocational opportunities, and a lack of theory and practice among career guidance teachers (13).

Against this background, a non-governmental organization attempted to incorporate the positive youth development approach in the design of a life and career development program for Secondary 3 students from a government-subsidized school within the context of the P.A.T.H.S. Project (14, 15). When the Secondary 3 students were facing the need to select subjects for the Hong Kong Diploma of Secondary Education Examination (HKDSE) and their genuine needs in life and career development, the principal and teachers of the school discovered anxiety and loss of direction in these students. With the collaboration of a non-governmental organization, a life and career development program using the positive youth development approach was launched in the secondary school during the academic years of 2013-2014, 2014-2015 and 2015-2016. The program aimed at developing the competencies of Secondary 3 students and motivating them in the formulation of life goals.

The program reported in this paper covered eight sessions. The first two sessions took a whole form approach to introduce the concepts of life career planning to the students and raise their awareness of the importance of life goal formulation. A talk and a workshop (the "mini society") were organized. The third to eighth sessions used a group-work strategy to provide different experiential opportunities for the participants to experience, reflect and learn. These programs included: a) adventure-based training program to build their resilience, problem-solving capacity and teamwork of the students, b) a workshop on understanding the life course of career development through experiential games, c) visits to enterprises and sharing sessions with entrepreneurs so as to understand the importance of life goal formulation and persistence attitudes, d) a simulated job interview for the students to realize the requirements of the employers and learn the expression skills, e) a "university hunt" to motivate the students in their life planning, and f) an award presentation ceremony to reinforce and award the students for their effort and participation. The Program was highly appreciated by the students (16). It is both interesting and important to extract the factors contributing to the success of the program as it is a novel attempt to integrate positive youth development paradigm and life career development intervention strategy in Hong Kong.

This study examined the factors contributing to the success of a life and career development program adopting the positive youth development approach that was delivered to secondary school students in Hong Kong. In the study, the chief program implementer and two cohorts of participants (2014-2015 and 2015-2016) were invited to share their views and experience after joining the program respectively. The focus group methodology was widely used in different phases and programs of the Project P.A.T.H.S. (17).

OUR STUDY

The data were collected from both implementer and participants. The chief program designer-cum-implementer of the Tier 2 Program of the Project P.A.T.H.S. during the academic years of 2014-2015 and 2015-2016 was invited for an in-depth interview. She was a social worker who had been working in a non-governmental organization for three years at the time of interview. Her main duty was to design, implement and coordinate Project P.A.T.H.S. in several schools, including the studied school. Informed consent of the social worker was sought. The interview was conducted by the researcher based on an interview guide (Appendix 1). The interview was conducted in a university and lasted for one hour and 30 minutes.

Besides, the participants of the Tier 2 Program of the Project P.A.T.H.S. (i.e., the life and career development program adopting the positive youth development approach) during the academic years of 2014-2015 and 2015-2016 were invited to participate in the study. They were Secondary 3 students in a government-subsidized secondary school. There were 36 and 35 students joining the programs in 2014-2015 and 2015-2016 respectively. All students were invited to participate in the focus groups, and 30 and 27 students from the two cohorts joined the focus groups respectively. Informed consent was obtained from both parents and students. Eight focus groups were formed within the two years.

The focus group interviews were conducted separately in different classrooms. The school social workers and program implementer assigned the students to different focus groups, with a balanced number of students between gender and class. There were around six to eight students in each group. The teachers and social workers did not stay in the classroom so that the students could talk more freely and openly. Each focus group was conducted by a trained researcher (i.e., the moderator of the focus group). The moderator conducted the focus group interview according to an interview guide (Appendix 2). The students were encouraged to share their experience and views of the Program. The focus group interviews lasted for one hour. All interviews were audio-recorded with the consent of the participants, and the verbatim was transcribed by the student helpers.

A general qualitative approach was employed in this study (18). Theme analyses pattern coding was performed to analyze the factors contributing to the success of the program (19). In principle, the broad themes were extracted from the transcripts of the verbatim.

OUR FINDINGS

Six themes were extracted from the transcripts of the verbatim, namely 1) clear objectives and strong emphasis on psychosocial development, 2) diverse and creative program design, 3) experiential approach so that the participants could experience, reflect and learn, 4) quality of implementers and instructors, 5) continuous feedback from the participants, and 6) good timing for the launch of the program. Each theme will be discussed in the following paragraphs.

Clear objectives and strong emphasis on psychosocial development

The non-governmental organization had prior experience in running life and career development programs, with a strong emphasis on enhancing adolescent psychosocial development. This facilitated the use of positive youth development approach in designing the Program. The paragraph below highlights a narrative of the implementer:

> Moderator: In what aspects do you think the life and career program in the Project P.A.T.H.S. enhances adolescent development?
> Implementer: Project P.A.T.H.S. contains different components of adolescent development. The life and career planning program helps the adolescents enhance their self-understanding, and build their positive self-identity. It is expected that the Program would help the adolescents explore their strengths and value systems, which is related to a clear self-identity. The Program also reminds the adolescents to be self-confident.

Another point is that the Program emphasizes how adolescents set their goals...their goals of their future. Throughout the Program, being aligned with the goal setting is the ability to make decisions, that means, the adolescents need to develop self-determination capacity so as to make a better choice for themselves.

Diverse and creative program design

The program design was innovative and diverse. The implementer and instructors meticulously designed the programs to meet the needs of the students:

> Implementer: We hope to provide a variety of programs for the students, especially more outings [outside activities] and adventure-based activities so that they can obtain more information from the outside, and gain more experience.

Though the Program covered only eight sessions, there were different activities provided to the students. The programs included simulation games, adventure-based training, visits to enterprises, sharing sessions with the entrepreneurs, a "university hunt" cum a sharing session with university students, simulated job interviews and an award presentation ceremony. The students' comments on each activity are listed below:

Simulation games
The simulation games were activities designed by the non-governmental organization to simulate the real-life situations of the work environment and the society. For instance, the "mini society" was a simulation game in which the participants were involved in the activities taking place in the society, such as passing the public examinations, finding jobs, earning a salary, investing the shares, and buying houses, etc. The participants learnt the rules and patterns of the operation of the society, and at the same time experienced the unexpected changes and chaos. The participants then

shared their experience and reflections after the games. The narratives below are some reflections of the students:

> Student A: I started to understand the importance of life planning. In the "mini society" game, it seemed that it was easy to perform the role, and I did not take it seriously. Eventually, I got bankrupt. And I totally lost all things. At that moment, I thought it was too difficult to be successful even in a game. In the real life, it was ten times more difficult. Not all things would run smoothly by themselves. Then I realized the importance of life planning. If I had not participated in the program, I would have never thought of life plans and I would be a termite of the society after graduation.

> Student B: I have impressive experience in the life and career workshop. In the game, the bank went bankrupt. At that time, I learnt that we have to be alert to what is happening in the society, and cannot just blindly follow others to obtain something, like money... Because of the greed, they invested a lot, and eventually went bankrupt.

> Student C: In the "mini society" game, because of my educational level, I was not entitled for a better job with a good prospect...When I realized that I could not earn adequate money to support my living, and failed to go to university, I was lost.

> Student D: After the "mini society" game, I realized that I could not only have dreams and nothing else. Even if you have dreams, you have to see whether you have the conditions to fulfil the dreams. That's why we need to have life goals and plans.

Adventure-based activities

The non-governmental organization provided a one-day adventure-based training for the students. The program aimed to build the team spirit and cooperation among the students, and develop their resilience and problem-solving capacities. The narratives below highlight the experience and reflections of the students after the activities.

Student E: In the adventure-based activity, I learnt to trust others. There was a high wall and we needed to climb over it. I thought it was more difficult than touching the sky.
Moderator: And you learnt to cooperate with others?
Student E: Yes.
Student F: It enhanced my self-confidence.
Moderator: Can you elaborate more?
Student F: Similar to Student E, when I climbed up the wall, I was very frightened. I have a phobia of heights. But the teammates raised me up. I didn't feel so frightened at that moment.
Moderator: Did other people help you?
Student F: Yes.
Student G: I learnt to be more active in problem-solving.
Moderator: Can you elaborate more?
Student G: Find ways. In the adventure-based program, we were in a team. We had to find ways to solve the problems. I shared my ideas on how we could solve the problems, and others also shared their views, and we modified our ideas together.

Visits to local enterprises and sharing of the entrepreneurs

The students had a chance to visit the enterprises and shared with the entrepreneurs. During 2014-2015, the students were arranged to visit a local hotel in Hong Kong and shared with the hotel manager. The students learnt more in the field of hospitality management. During 2015-2016, the students paid a visit to a local café in Hong Kong and shared with the owner. Also, they attended a leather product-making workshop and shared with the entrepreneur. The students were inspired by the spirit of entrepreneurship. The narratives below are some reflections from the students:

> Student H: I knew more about the job market. For instance, the hotel manager shared his work experience with us, and introduced the hospitality industry to us…This reminded me to think over what jobs I would choose in the future, and which subjects I should select.

Student I: In the visit to the cafe, the owner started his business by himself. His socio-economic background was not good at that time. But he succeeded. Now he has two cafes. He gave me courage to pursue my own dream.

Student J: In the handmade leather product workshop, not only I learnt how to use the leather to make different products, but also the instructor shared with us her experience, that is, we have to formulate our life goals.

"University hunt" and sharing of university students

Using the adventure-based training approach, a visit to a university was modified as a program of "university hunt" to understand the university life. The students were asked to search for different checkpoints and to complete the assigned task at each checkpoint. Most of the tasks required the students to work together and approach the university students to share their university life. Furthermore, a visit to a student hostel and sharing with university students were arranged. The narratives below highlight the experience and reflections from the students:

Student L: I like the program of "University Hunt". My aspiration is to study in university. I obtained more information from the program, especially the university life. My classmates and I were particularly curious about the hall life...We also had a sharing session with the university students... about the curriculum, learning study life...My parents told me that the university life was the happiest time in the learning path. I also hope to experience that... In the program, I had a chance to experience as a university student. Our instructor provided a Powerpoint presentation in a lecture room, and I felt like having a lecture in the university.

Moderator: What did you learn in the program?

Student L: I learnt that we need to plan well so as to be admitted to the university.

Simulated job interviews
Steps of job application were introduced to the students. Students were requested to select a job and write their resume. A simulated job interview was arranged for each student. Feedback was given on the performance of the students. Moreover, the students also performed the role of interviewer in the other classmates' interviews. By taking a reciprocal role, they learnt more on the seniors' expectation of recruiting new staff. The narratives below are the experience of a student:

> Student M: Before the job interviews, the instructor told us that we had to undertake three steps. The first is that you have to search what kind of jobs that you would like to apply. The second one is to write your resume. The last one is the job interview. We were assigned to different groups. We did the job interviews in different rooms. On top of the instructor, two students also performed the role of interviewer. And finally they gave me feedback.
> Moderator: What kind of job did you apply?
> Student M: Salesman.
> Moderator: What did you learn in the experience?
> Student M: To have eye contact. When they ask you questions, you have to respond tactfully.

Experiential learning approach – students learnt from participation and experience

Experiential learning approach was adopted in the Program. Students were required to participate in the activities and learnt from experience. Self-reflection and mutual sharing of the experience are crucial for the students to consolidate what they have learnt in the activities. The narratives below are the description of the implementer on the use of experiential learning approach.

> Moderator: What are the special features of the Program?

Implementer: I think that the Program contains diverse programs for the students. Some were implemented in school, and some brought the students outside the school and let them experience. Compared to the programs that only provide information to the students, this Program would make more changes in the students. It is because after the students experienced from the activities that they haven't tried before, they reflected on the [new] experience and listened to others' sharing. This is the real experience that they have, which is different from the materials that our agency or social workers "would impose" on them. I believe that this type of learning would generate more changes in the students.

The students were impressed and benefited from participating in the activities and consolidating their experience through reflections. The narratives below highlight the views of the students.

Student N: It is different from the previous programs that were conducted in school. Majority of the [previous] programs were that we sat down and listened to the speaker. But in this program, we gained experience on our own. True, we taste it by ourselves, and get in touch of our future. The materials and information made me feel clear about my future.

Student O: They really allowed us to experience by ourselves. For instance, in the program of the "university hunt", they let us explore on campus and find out the answers. And in the "mini society", they let us choose our life paths.

Orientation and quality of implementers

The positive orientation and quality of the implementers constituted greatly to the success of the Program. The implementers had clear roles as program leaders. They focused mainly on the psychosocial development instead of vocational preparation of the students. They maintained good interactions with the students.

Clear role identification

The implementers focused mainly on the psychosocial development instead of vocational preparation of the students, as described by the narratives of the implementer:

> Implementer: When talking about the needs of the students, in fact, I emphasize intrapersonal development of adolescents. This relates greatly to their academic performance, and their lives. How do the students perceive their self-identity? How do they plan for their life paths? This is the stage that they need to explore their lives. I, as an adult, need to give them right principles and positive attitudes, and enhance their vigor to make their own decisions and try them out. I think adolescents need to develop themselves.
>
> Moderator: Can you share with us some of your consolidated experience in conducting this type of program?
>
> Implementer: An important consideration is how we assess the needs of the students. The school approached us for life and career planning [program] as they discovered the needs of the students. You may know that the students were studying in Secondary 3. If you do walk in their shoes, what are the students' needs? Except the core need that the students have to choose their subjects for DSE, are there any other students' needs that the school seldom explores? Having adequate resources [provided by Project P.A.T.H.S.], we hoped to provide some new experience to the students that they have never had.

Strengths-based orientation

Echoing the positive youth development paradigm of P.A.T.H.S., the implementers adopted the strengths-based perspective to understand the students and enhance their competencies:

> Moderator: How do you describe the adolescents nowadays?
>
> Implementer: The adolescents nowadays... I think they also want to make changes. They are a group of adolescents looking for changes. They have many creative and independent ideas, but many of them do not know how to express themselves.

Caring role of the implementers

The implementers emphasized the "peer" role in engaging and interacting with the students, which resulted in a supportive, caring and egalitarian implementer-participant relationship. The narratives below highlight the views of the implementer.

> Moderator: How do you describe your relationship with the students?
> Implementer: Relationship with the students? It is positive. Although I am an implementer, I hope to take a "peer" role to share with the students... Still I had something that I insisted, such as the communication styles of the students and the program safety. I stood firm on these parts as these were related to the safety and politeness of the students. Other than these, I used a peer role to share with the students what they cared about, such as the university life. If the content did not go beyond some basic principles, I liked to share my experiences with them, hoping that they would understand more. I think this is why we can maintain a good positive relationship...I think [the attitude] to treat the students is a sense of mutual respect.

In fact, the students appreciated the care and support from the implementers. The narratives below show their appreciation of the implementers.

> Student P: The instructor cared much about our future. On the way we left the hotel, she shared her experience with us of her aspiration when she was young. She told me that she wanted to be a hotel manager. But she found that hospitality management did not match her well, and thus she finally chose social work. Another instructor shared that she actually tried out a hotel manager, and shared her job experience to me.
> Moderator: How did this affect you?
> Student P: In the beginning, I did not expect that they did care about my future, and would share with me...But after that, I found that the program affected me a lot. They [the instructors] really cared about us. They worked hard for us, and let us understand ourselves and know more about different jobs. They did not want to see that we chose the jobs that we did not prefer at all.

Student Q: They [the instructors] were very pleasant. They always smiled and shared with us nicely. Though sometimes we were tired and snoozed, they never scolded us, just reminded us with a smile. I appreciate that.

Responsible and devoted implementers
The students were impressed by the implementers' effort to design and implement the Program. The implementers also performed as good role models for the students to learn and imitate. The narratives below highlight the views of the students:

Student R: I found that all implementers [of the program] meticulously designed the programs for us, and I learnt a lot in the programs.

Student S: They [the implementers] were very devoted. They explained the information in detail. For example, the four steps of life and career planning…They always reminded us of these.

Student T: They [the implementers] were very attentive. They made a great effort to prepare the materials for us. This really influenced me. I may need to be attentive in my work, and never do things carelessly.

Continuous feedback from the students

The implementers constantly consulted the school teachers and students, and collected feedback from the students. The visits to the hotel and cafe were the results of suggestions of the teachers and students. This also reflected the egalitarian relationship and mutual respect among the implementers, school teachers and the students.

Implementer: [We] continuously collected feedback from the students and then modified and adjusted our programs.

Good timing – students need to select subjects for DSE

Secondary 3 students were ready to participate in the life and career development program as they needed to select subjects for the Hong Kong Diploma of Secondary Education Examination (DSE). The students were misted in the selection of subjects as they understood that the selection was critical in their study and thus their future, yet they seldom thought of their life plans. The selection of subjects acted as a catalyst for the students to join the Program and think over their life goals. The narratives below are the reflections of the students:

> Student U: Secondary 3 is a turning point. We need to know what is happening in our society. This would affect me. The Program helped me to find out my life goals, and the aspects that I need to explore more.

> Student V: When I studied in Secondary 3, I found great changes in the curriculum between Secondary 2 and 3. And we have to select subjects (for DSE) at the end of the academic year. I had difficulties in doing it in a short period of time. I really did not know what was suitable for me. But after the program (life and career workshop) and going outside, I have more understanding of the outside world. I have some threads of what is suitable for me… I hope to make a right choice.
> Moderator: What is the largest impact of the Program?
> Student V: I start to think seriously about what I want to do in the future, that is, what I dream to do and my life goals. In the past, I was lost. I really did not know what was happening. But time flies. After the Program, I start to think over my dream and life goals.

DISCUSSION

The study explored the factors that contributed to the success of a life and career planning program adopting a positive youth development approach from the perspectives of implementers and students. The factors comprised the hardware and software of the Program in promoting adolescent psychosocial competence and motivating them in life goal formulation. The hardware included the use of positive youth development approach in orientating and designing the Program, which reaffirmed the enhancement of psychosocial competence to be the main objective of life and career development. This also aligns with the essence of life career development that focuses on the development of life competencies, attitudes and values of individuals (20). Furthermore, the meticulous design of the program content, and the diverse and creative programs (such as simulation games, university hunt, adventure-based training, visits to the enterprises) also contributed to the hardware. These programs allowed dynamic interaction among the students, and between the students and other people. The programs also employed the experiential learning strategy (21) in the implementation. Experiential learning involves four stages: concrete experience, reflective observation, abstract conceptualization, and active experimentation (21). The Program allowed the students to experience through participating in the activities. They reflected on their actions and reactions in the activities and shared their experience with other teammates, which in turn enhanced their self-understanding. When the students realized the importance of abstract concepts of life planning and positive youth development, they got the insights and tried out the new concepts in the real-life practice.

However, the Program would never succeed without the software. The software was the positive orientation and qualities of the implementers. They were the ones who engaged the students in the activities, passed the messages on to the students and acted as the change agent in the intervention process. Hence, it is essential for the implementers to have a clear orientation on the purpose and focus of life and career development, and hold positive angles on the strengths and potential of the adolescents. In the previous phases of the Program, adventure-based counseling has been shown to promote holistic youth development (22).

There are several theoretical and practical implications of the present findings. In the face of criticism that life and career development takes a peripheral role in motivating adolescents in search of life goals, and focuses mainly on information dissemination (13), this Program serves as an exemplar of using positive youth development paradigm in the design and implementation of life and career development program, and this is novel in the practice. As suggested by Savickas et al. (23), the framework of career counseling and interventions should be life-long, holistic, contextual and preventive. Positive youth development approach that emphasizes adolescents' strengths, potential and competencies will serve as a constructive theoretical framework of the life and career development.

Practically, the study suggested the importance of the quality and orientation of the implementers to the success of a life and career program. In secondary schools, the career guidance personnel are the crucial persons who design, implement and monitor the life and career development programs in school. It is essential to equip them with a holistic positive youth development paradigm as well as the theoretical models of life and career development. Moreover, the career guidance personnel may need to take up more a caring role in engaging their students, and develop a trusting teacher-student relationship. Furthermore, the experiential learning approach increases the students' motivation and facilitates their learning through experience, reflection and sharing. The career guidance personnel may need to provide more experiential learning opportunities for the students to explore their career. Last but not least, the schools may need to cultivate a life-long and holistic orientation on adolescent development across all disciplines, and ensure that the teachers understand the primary focus of life and career development.

There are several limitations of the study. First, the findings were based on the qualitative data collected from one secondary school in Hong Kong. The school environment may be influential in determining the success of the Program. It is advised that the Program in other schools would be replicated and related evaluation studies would be conducted. Second, focus group interviews were conducted at one time point, i.e., in the last session of the Program. It is suggested that ongoing qualitative evaluation of the Program would be conducted. Third, peer checking and member checking were not performed due to the time and manpower constraints, and these may reduce the creditability of the study (18).

Despite the limitations, the study examined the successful factors of a life and career planning program using a positive youth development approach implemented in a secondary school in Hong Kong. It provides insights for educators, researchers and social workers into the further development of life and career planning in the context of Hong Kong.

ACKNOWLEDGMENTS

The Project P.A.T.H.S. and preparation for this paper were financially supported by The Hong Kong Jockey Club Charities Trust. This paper is based on an article published in the International Journal on Disability and Human Development 2018;17(3) issue. We thank the participants for joining this study.

APPENDIX 1. INTERVIEW GUIDE OF THE INTERVIEW OF IMPLEMENTER

Program's rationale, ideas and framework

- How do you describe the needs and situations of Hong Kong adolescents nowadays?
- Do you agree with the rationale and framework of Project P.A.T.H.S.? Which parts do you agree? Which parts do you disagree?
- How did you design the framework and content of the life and career development program?
- How did you link up positive youth development and life and career planning?
- What do you think life and career planning is more related with the constructs of positive youth development?

- How did you demonstrate the constructs of positive youth development in the life and career planning program?

Effectiveness of the Program

- To what extent did the Tier 2 program of Project P.A.T.H.S. help the psychosocial development of the participants? Please give some examples on your views.
- Did you find any changes in the participants after they joined the Project? If yes, what are the changes?
- In case there were changes in the participants, what are the factors that you perceive contributing to the changes?
- Did the changes meet the objectives?
- What were the intervention strategies that induced the changes?
- In case there were no changes in the participants, what are the reasons that you perceive?

The implementation of the Program

- In the implementation of the Tier 2 program of Project P.A.T.H.S., what were the responses of the students in general? Can you give some examples?
- Can you share some of your experience and techniques for implementing the Program (such as training skills, instructor-participant relationships)?
- Did you have any difficulties in implementing the Tier 2 program of Project P.A.T.H.S.? If yes, please share some examples. How did you solve them?
- What are the features of the Program? Please give some examples to support your views.
- Do you think that the Program is a successful one? Please state your reasons.

- Based on your experience of conducting the Tier 2 program of Project P.A.T.H.S., what things should the implementers bear in mind?

Overall comments

- Overall, how do you comment on the approach of the Tier 2 program of Project P.A.T.H.S.?
- What is your overall impression of the Program? Did you enjoy it?

APPENDIX 2. INTERVIEW GUIDE OF THE FOCUS GROUP FOR PARTICIPANTS

Experience of students' participation in the program

- How did you realize this program? How did you enroll in the program?
- What were your expectations before you joined the program? From a retrospective view, how far did the program fulfill your expectations?
- In the program, which part did you like the most? Why?
- In the program, which part did you dislike the most? Why?
- Can you share an occasion/event that you think very impressive? What makes this occasion/event to be the most impressive one? What do you learn from the experience?
- Do you think you are involved in the program? Why or why not?

Comments on the program process

- What are your comments on the instructors?
- What are your relationships with the instructors? Do you feel friendly with them?

- Did you know the groupmates before the program?
- Did you have any changes in the relationships with your groupmates? If yes, what are the changes?

Comments on the program effectiveness

- What do you benefit the most from the program?
- Did you have any changes after participating in the program? If yes, what are the changes? What makes you have the changes?
- Do you think the program has helped your development? If yes, what are they?
- Do you think the program has helped your adjustment in your school life? If yes, what are they?

Overall comments

- Overall, what do you appreciate the most in the program?
- Do you have any suggestions on how the program can be improved?
- If you are invited to use three descriptors to describe the program, what three words will you use?

REFERENCES

[1] Twenge JM. Generation ME: Why today's young Americans are more confident, assertive, entitled - and more miserable than ever before. New York: Free Press, 2006.

[2] Tapscott D. Growing up digital: The rise of the net generation. New York: McGraw-Hill, 1998.

[3] Howe N, Strauss W. Millennials rising: The next generation. New York: Vintage Books, 2000.

[4] Schneider B, Stevenson D. The ambitious generation: America's teenagers, motivated but directionless. New Haven: Yale University Press, 1999.

[5] Engels DW, editor. The professional practice of career counseling and consultation: A resource document, 2nd ed. Alexandria, VA: American Counseling Association, 1994.

[6] Lapan RT, Adams A, Turner S, Hinkelman JM. Seventh graders vocational interest and efficacy expectation patterns. J Career Dev 2000;26:215-29.

[7] Zhang W, Hu X, Pope M. The evolution of career guidance and counseling in the People's Republic of China. Career Dev Q 2002;50(3):226-36.

[8] Solberg VS, Howard KA, Blustein DL, Close W. Career development in the schools connecting school-to-work-to-life. Couns Psychol 2002;30(5):705-25.

[9] Sue D, Sue DW, Sue D, Sue S. Essentials of understanding abnormal behavior, 2nd ed. Belmont, CA: Wadsowrth Cengage Learning, 2014.

[10] Damon W. What is positive youth development? Ann Am Acad Pol Soc Sci 2004;591:13-24.

[11] Shek DTL, Siu AMH, Lee TY. The Chinese Positive Youth Development Scale: A validation study. Res Soc Work Pract 2007;17:380-91.

[12] Career Guidance Section, Education Bureau. Life planning education and career guidance for secondary schools, 1st ed. Hong Kong: Career Guidance Section, School Development Division, Education Bureau, 2014. URL: https://careerguidance.edb.hkedcity.net/edb/export/sites/default/lifeplanning/.pdf/about-careers-guidance/CLP-Guide_full_E.pdf.

[13] Leung SA. Career counseling in Hong Kong: Meeting the social challenges. Career Dev Q 2002;50(3):237-45.

[14] Shek DTL, Merrick J, eds. Special issue: Positive youth development and training. London: Freund, 2010.

[15] Shek DTL, Sun RCF, Merrick J, eds. Positive youth development: Theory, research and application. New York: Nova Science, 2013.

[16] Leung JTY, Shek DTL. Perceived benefits of a life and career development program adopting positive youth development approach in Hong Kong. Int J Child Adolesc Health, in press.

[17] Shek DTL. The use of focus groups in programme evaluation: Experience based on the Project P.A.T.H.S. in a Chinese context. In: Barbour RS, Morgan DL, eds. A new era in focus group research. Hampshire: Palgrave Macmillan, in press.

[18] Shek DTL, Tang VMY, Han XY. Evaluation of evaluation studies using qualitative research methods in the social work literature (1990-2003): Evidence that constitutes a wake-up call. Res Soc Work Pract 2005;15(3):180-94.

[19] Miles MB, Huberman AM. Qualitative data analysis. Thousand Oaks, CA: Sage, 1994.

[20] Gysbers NC, Moore EJ. Beyond career development – Life career development. Pers Guid J 1975;53(9):647-54.

[21] Kolb DA. Experiential learning: Experience as the source of learning and development. Englewood Cliffs, NJ: Prentice-Hall, 1984.

[22] Shek DTL, Lee TY. Helping adolescents with greater psychosocial needs: Subjective outcome evaluation based on different cohorts. ScientificWorldJournal 2012;2012:Article ID 694018. DOI: 10.1100/2012/694018
[23] Savickas ML, Nota L, Rossier J, Dauwalder JP, Duarte ME, Guichard J, et al. Life designing: A paradigm for career construction in the 21st century. J Vocat Behav 2009;75(3):239-50.

In: Psychosocial Needs
Editors: Daniel TL Shek et al.

ISBN: 978-1-53611-951-0
© 2017 Nova Science Publishers, Inc.

Chapter 7

PERCEIVED BENEFITS OF A LIFE AND CAREER DEVELOPMENT PROGRAM

Janet TY Leung[1,*]*, PhD*
and Daniel TL Shek[1-5]*, PhD, FHKPS, BBS, SBS, JP*

[1]Department of Applied Social Sciences,
The Hong Kong Polytechnic University, Hong Kong, PR China
[2]Centre for Innovative Programmes for Adolescents and Families,
The Hong Kong Polytechnic University, Hong Kong, PR China,
[3]Department of Social Work, East China Normal University,
Shanghai, PR China
[4]Kiang Wu Nursing College of Macau, Macau, PR China
[5]Division of Adolescent Medicine, Department of Pediatrics,
Kentucky Children's Hospital,
University of Kentucky College of Medicine, Lexington,
Kentucky, US

---

[*] Correspondence: Janet Leung, PhD, Department of Applied Social Sciences, The Hong Kong Polytechnic University, Hunghom, Hong Kong, PR China. Email: janet.leung@polyu.edu.hk.

In this chapter we present a qualitative evaluation study which examined the subjective experience and perceived benefits of 57 Secondary 3 students who had participated in a life and career development project using the positive youth development approach in a Tier 2 Program of the Project P.A.T.H.S. in Hong Kong. Focus group methodology was adopted in the study. Results showed that the students had very positive views about the program. They expressed that the program enhanced their intrapersonal competence (self-confidence, courage, resilience and future aspirations) as well as interpersonal competence (cooperation and communication skills of the students through teamwork). The students had reflections of their past lifestyles and were motivated to make positive changes. They became more forward-looking on their future paths, and showed eagerness to establish their life goals, formulate their future plans, and research more information on their future aspirations. The present study provides evidence on the effectiveness of the use of positive youth development programs in nurturing the holistic development of Chinese adolescents through life and career development programs.

INTRODUCTION

"What do you want to be in the future?" is a question that most of us encountered when we were young. Different occupations such as policeman, teacher, farmer, doctor, nurse, etc. have appeared in the compositions and drawings of the kids. As expected, people may change their occupational aspirations when they grow up and acquire more knowledge about the nature of different careers, information on the changing world, as well as self-understanding about their personalities, interests and competencies (1, 2). As such, the developmental task of "career" seems to accompany us in our development.

Career is the "time extended working out of a purposeful life pattern through work undertaken by the person" (3, p.6). Based on Super's lifespan-life space approach of career (2, 4), an individual undergoes different stages of career development in compliance with the personal life-span development. In each stage, one may need to fulfill the life and career tasks so as to transit to another stage. During the stage of adolescence, one may transit from the growth stage to the exploration stage, which is characterized by the development of one's self-concept in terms of competence, interests, attitudes and needs. Hence, positive youth development is critical to adolescents in their life and career development, and the positive youth development attributes are the building blocks of the future career competencies of an individual. This also echoes the trait-factors theory (5) that posits the importance of congruence between one's personal styles and the occupational environment. Indeed, self-understanding is crucial for identifying the personal traits of an individual.

Gysbers and colleagues (6, 7) expanded the ideas of career development to include life development. Life career development is defined as "self-development over the life span through the integration of the roles, settings, and events of a person's life" (6 p. 648). Rather than taking a narrow perspective of "vocational development" and "career counseling", life career development takes a more comprehensive perspective to integrate human development across the life span (2). Hence, life and career development enhances the development of life competencies, attitudes and values so that an individual can master his/her own life.

From this point of view, life and career development aligns with the concepts of positive youth development. Positive youth development emphasizes the importance of assets, strengths and competencies of adolescents (8, 9). Benson (10) identified 40 developmental assets. Lerner et al. (11) identified six "C"s of positive youth development, namely competence, confidence, connection, character, caring and contribution. Catalano et al. (12) proposed a systematic framework of adolescent positive youth development and highlighted fifteen positive youth development constructs, namely bonding, resilience, cognitive competence, emotional competence, moral competence, behavioral competence, social competence, spirituality, beliefs in the future, clear and positive identity, self-determination, self-efficacy, prosocial involvement, prosocial norms and recognition of positive behavior. The competency-building paradigm provides a strong conceptual framework for the design of a life and career development program.

This study examined the perceived benefits of the participants who joined a life and career development project using the positive youth development approach under the Project P.A.T.H.S. (Positive Adolescent Training through Holistic Social Programmes). The Project P.A.T.H.S. adopts the positive youth development approach to implement a large-scale positive youth development program for junior secondary school students (i.e., Grades 7 to 9) in Hong Kong. There are two tiers in the Project. Tier 1 Program is a structural universal curriculum to enhance psychosocial competencies of all junior secondary school students, whereas Tier 2 Program targets students with greater psychosocial needs and makes use of diverse intervention strategies in helping the adolescents enhance their interpersonal and intrapersonal development. In the past few years, the majority of Tier 2 Programs employed adventure-based counseling and voluntary services as the core program design (13, 14). There is empirical evidence showing that Tier 2 Programs were effective in helping the adolescents develop their competencies (13-15).

The program reported in this paper adhered to the positive youth development paradigm of the Project P.A.T.H.S. and used a life and career development strategy to provide different learning opportunities for adolescents to develop their psychosocial competencies. The program aimed at developing the competencies and motivation of Secondary 3 students in their search of life goals and career development. The program covered eight sessions. The first two sessions took a whole form approach to introduce the concepts of life career planning to the students and increase their awareness of the importance of life goal formulation. The third to eighth sessions used a group-work strategy to provide different experiential opportunities for the participants to experience, reflect and learn. These programs included: a) adventure-based training program, b) an experiential life workshop; c) a visit to an enterprise and a sharing session with an entrepreneur, d) a simulated job interview for the students, e) a university hunt and a sharing session with university students, and f) an award presentation ceremony. Table 1 lists the objectives, nature and program details of the Project during the academic years of 2014-2015 and 2015-2016.

Table 1. Program content

	Program session	Objectives	Capacity	2014 Program	2015 Program
1	Talk on life and career development	• To arouse interest of the students on life and career development • To build up students' knowledge on concepts of life and career development	All Secondary 3 students	• Talk on concepts of life and career development	• Talk on concepts of life and career development
2	Workshop on life and career development	• To arouse interest of the students on life and career development • To enhance students' understanding on the importance of life and career planning	All Secondary 3 students	• Experiential exercise: The mini society	• Experiential exercise: The mini society
3	Adventure-based training	• To enhance resilience and problem-solving skills of the students • To build up team cohesion of the group	A group of Secondary 3 students	• Day camp	• Day camp
4	Advanced training workshop on life and career development	• To enhance self-understanding of the students • To introduce the life course of career development • To motivate the students on life goal formulation	A group of Secondary 3 students	• Advanced workshop on life and career development – experiential games	• Advanced workshop on life and career development – experiential games

Table 1. (Continued)

	Program session	Objectives	Capacity	2014 Program	2015 Program
5	Exposure program – a visit to an enterprise	• To let students learn from the experience of others on entrepreneurship • To motivate the students on life goal formulation	A group of Secondary 3 students	• A visit to a local hotel and interview with the hotel manager	• A visit to a local cafe and interview with the cafe owner • Workshop of a hand-made leather production and interview with the owner-cum-instructor
6	Job interview workshop	• To build the expression skills and confidence of the students • To enhance the students' self-motivation	A group of Secondary 3 students	• Experiential exercise: Job application and interview	• Experiential exercise: Job application and interview
7	Exposure program – the university hunt	• To enhance the problem-solving skills of the students • To let students get familiar with the university life • To motivate the students on life goal formulation	A group of Secondary 3 students	• A visit to a university and an adventure-based university hunt	• A visit to a university and an adventure-based university hunt
8	Graduation ceremony	• To reinforce and award the students for their effort and participation • To conduct program evaluation	A group of Secondary 3 students	• Award presentation and program evaluation	• Award presentation and program evaluation

This chapter reports the perceived benefits of the participants who participated in the aforementioned life and career development project using the positive youth development approach in Tier 2 Program of the Project P.A.T.H.S. Focus group interview strategy was employed in the study. Focus group is defined as "a qualitative research technique used to obtain data about feelings and opinions of a small group of participants about a given problem, experience, service or other phenomenon" (16, p. 414). Focus group is a useful and effective strategy to capture the views, ideas and experiences of the participants (17). As Kitzinger (18) suggested that focus group "capitalises on communication between research participants in order to generate data" (18, p. 299), this data collection strategy allows communication among participants to generate more ideas and rich content on the topic. The focus group methodology has been extensively used in the Project P.A.T.H.S. in the past years (19).

OUR RESEARCH

The data were collected from the participants of the Tier 2 Program of the Project P.A.T.H.S. (i.e., life and career development program using the positive youth development approach) during the academic years of 2014-2015 and 2015-2016. They were Secondary 3 students in a government-subsidized secondary school. There were 36 and 35 students joining the programs in 2014-2015 and 2015-2016 respectively. All students were invited to participate in the focus groups. Informed consent was obtained from both parents and students. Finally, 30 and 27 students joined the focus groups in the two cohorts respectively, forming a total of eight focus groups in the study.

The focus group interviews were conducted separately in different classrooms. In each cohort, the students were assigned to four focus groups based on their gender and class. There were six to eight students in each group. No other adults, except the trained researcher (i.e., the moderator of the focus group), were invited to join the focus group in order to allow students to talk more freely and openly. The moderator conducted the focus group interview according to an interview guide (Appendix 1). The students were encouraged to share their views and experiences of the program. The focus group interviews lasted for around an hour. All interviews were audio-recorded with the consent of the participants, and the verbatim was transcribed by the student helpers.

A general qualitative approach was employed in this study (20). Qualitative findings of the comments on the program effectiveness (i.e., Part 3 of the interview guide) were analyzed using theme analysis and pattern coding (21). The broad themes were extracted from the transcripts of the verbatim. Furthermore, the themes were further matched with the 15 positive youth development constructs highlighted in the Project P.A.T.H.S. (9).

Moreover, the responses to the last question "If you are invited to use three descriptors to describe the program, what three words will you use?" (Part 4: Overall comment) were also analyzed. The descriptors used by the students to describe the program were categorized into "positive," "neutral" and "negative" responses. This would give us an overview of how the students perceived the program.

OUR FINDINGS

Table 2 shows the responses of the students on the perceived benefits of the life and career development project using positive youth development constructs. It is not surprising to find that students showed enhancement in self-efficacy (e.g., researching more information for life goal formulation and making future plans), spirituality (e.g., setting clear and unswerving goals) and cognitive competence (e.g., more understanding of job nature and entrepreneurship), as these were the important elements of life and career development. From the sharing of Student A and Student B, they reviewed their lifestyles in the past and realized the importance of life goal formulation and planning for the future.

Table 2. Responses of the students on their perceived benefits from the project

Positive Youth Development Construct	Responses	Frequency	Examples of the Narratives
Beliefs in the future	Be optimistic about the future	2	• I find myself more optimistic about the future…I like to make leather products. But someone told me that I could not earn a living from that …I was lost about my future. But this time, the instructor [from the leather product workshop] shared her stories about entrepreneurship…She managed to fulfill her dream… The most important thing is whether you find a job that you like most, and feel satisfied with the job.
Cognitive competence	Know more about job nature and entrepreneurship	8	• Before joining the program, I know nothing about job seeking and entrepreneurship. After joining the program, I know more about different jobs. Then I feel less anxious.
	Be conscientious in your work	4	• You have to do the things with conscientiousness. If I do things in a "hea" [not conscientious] manner, I would lose the opportunities.
	Know more about the selection of subjects	4	• The Program helped me understand more about my future career and what subjects I should select…We have to plan even when we are in secondary school. We need to choose the subjects that we are interested in.
	Make better judgement with more information	1	• I understand more about the external environment. Then I will find out what is suitable for me and what is not. I can make better judgement.
	Increase creativity	1	• This made me become more creative.
Behavioral competence	Be diligent in study	14	• We must be diligent from now on. If we were not diligent, we could not find a good job in the future.

Table 2. (Continued)

Positive Youth Development Construct	Responses	Frequency	Examples of the Narratives
Behavioral competence	Be diligent in study	14	• In the past, I found that "happiness" was the most important thing, and I did not think of how I could enter the university… Now, I need to study hard…This will change my future.
	Self-discipline	2	• After listening to the sharing of the university students on how they manage themselves…I learn [the importance of] self-management even if no one monitors you.
	Increase the skills of job interview	4	• They taught you how to attend a job interview… how to respond to the questions and be polite … I learnt the basic principles of attending a job interview, and would not be innocent in the interview.
Self-efficacy	Make plans for the future	18	• I found the program enhanced my capacity to plan for the future. • I have a dream, and I decide what I need to do in the future…But now I need to research more my chosen occupation and my selected university, etc…I need to gather more information about the future, and make myself clearer [in my future plan].
	Be more active	2	• I waited for someone to tell me what to do [in the past]. But now, I become active to find the way out.
	Become more courageous	5	• I find myself more courageous. I used to be timid in the past.
Spirituality	Understand the purpose of life	2	• What we treasure in life is not wealth or money. Happy and simple life is fine.
	Set up clear and unswerving goals	12	• I think each person should have an unswerving goal. We should not change [the goals] too frequently. For example, you want to be a teacher, and then you want to be a chef. Then you will waste your effort. Therefore, I think we need to have a consistent goal so that we can fulfill our dream.

Perceived benefits of a life and career development program 131

Positive Youth Development Construct	Responses	Frequency	Examples of the Narratives
	Develop your interest and find your dream	5	• I will develop your interest, and find my dream.
	Find a direction and follow your dream	4	• I started to follow my dream [in my future plan].
Resilience	Get out from the challenges	2	• When we face adversity, we can think that the situation may not be so bad, that means we can think how to solve the problems. We need not keep thinking on the bad situations. We need to be optimistic.
	Be adaptive to different situations	1	• In case you are in a different environment, you must learn the attitudes to adapt to different situations.
	Prepare alternatives to prevent things from getting worse	1	• You need to see what you want to do in the future, and keep in mind that there may be unexpected scenarios. I need to prepare for the worst and find another way out.
Self-determination	Choose a suitable job	1	• When we grow up, we have to make a lot of choices. But how can we make a choice for a suitable job? ...We have to consider many possibilities.
Clear and positive identity	More mature	6	• I become more mature... I search for the materials from the website of the Labour Department... [In the simulation exercise] when I saw the job requirement, I found myself innocent...I did not meet the requirement... This inspired me to study hard in the future.
	Enhance leadership	2	• The program enhanced our leadership... as we can achieve a breakthrough together.
	Increase self-confidence	10	• I have confidence to tell my classmates why I want to do that job in the simulated job interview. • I become more confident...I was shy in the past.

Table 2. (Continued)

Positive Youth Development Construct	Responses	Frequency	Examples of the Narratives
	Understand my weaknesses	1	• I become more aware of my weaknesses, and I need to make improvement on them…I was a silly person in the past.
	Enhance self-understanding	2	• I know more about myself… through the psychological assessment.
Emotional competence	Become happier	2	• I become happier and less depressed than before as I always stayed at home in the past.
	Enhance empathy	1	• I start to understand other people's feelings.
Moral competence	Courage to admit wrong deeds	1	• When I was young, I did things without thinking of the consequences. But after joining the program, I know that I have to bear the consequences for my deeds. For instance, when I am wrong, I should admit it, and should not deny.
	Think of consequences before you act	2	• In the past, I was impulsive in doing things…and would not consider other people and the consequences. After joining the Program, I learnt to consider whether my actions would affect others and those I did not know.
Social competence	Enhance teamwork	7	• We need to have teamwork even if you own the business. You need others to help you and serve your business, and you should treat them well as a team…Teamwork, we started to learn in the adventure-based training program…If we have team spirit, we can achieve a breakthrough in the difficulties. • If you fail, the team would fail. In case we need to be successful, we need to work together.
	Cooperate with others	9	• The program enhanced my cooperation with others. In the tour to the university, we were divided into different groups. We needed to discuss, play and complete the tasks together. I learnt to be cooperative.

Perceived benefits of a life and career development program 133

Positive Youth Development Construct	Responses	Frequency	Examples of the Narratives
	Enhance communication skills	13	• I learnt how to communicate with those who I was not familiar with… The instructor deliberately separated those who always played together and assigned them to different groups. • I was introverted in Secondary 1 and 2… When I talked to others, I was just like talking to myself…I was afraid to talk to others…Now I am bolder.
	Trust other people	5	• I learnt to trust others, and this made us more united.
	Understand the roles	1	• I understand my roles and know how to support others.
Bonding	Enhance relationship with peers	2	• My relationship with my classmates is improved.
	Seek help from friends	1	• I learn to seek help from my friends. They will help me and bear my load.

"We have to cherish the time. The time of our secondary school life is short. Only six years; it flies in the blink of an eye. I do not want to feel regretful after six years. I have to cherish the six years and develop myself. After joining the program, I understand more about myself. I am different from who I was in Secondary 1 and 2. I used to play and relax after finishing my homework at that time. Now, I have to take action. After joining the program, I know more about myself. I start to formulate my life goals. I must make good use of these three years to set my goals and make plans…I hope I can achieve my goals through actions. Otherwise, after graduating from the secondary school, I might still get lost." (Student A)

"After joining the program, I find myself more mature. In the past, I always had this thought: 'what subjects to select (for DSE)? I can decide later'. But in fact, time is running so fast and we will be in Secondary 4. Subject selection is very important to me. I now learn it. I become more active in planning [my future]." (Student B)

At the same time, students showed that the program enhanced their self-confidence and psychological maturity, promoted their diligence in their study and built up their courage. The Project also enhanced the wellbeing of the students. The paragraphs below were some students' reflections on their changes:

> "I am a person who easily gets stressed. But I am better than the previous 'me'. In the past, I felt stressed whenever I handled different tasks, and was frightened that I could not complete them. But after joining the Project, I become more confident. When I face a new task, I am firm to say, 'Good, I can do it'. I am not as hesitant as before." (Student C)

> "I become less passive [after joining the program]. When there are activities, I will join. I learn more and play more...After joining this program, I found myself happier. It's different from the past when I was depressed and always stayed at home. After participating in a series of activities, I would attempt to gain more experience. I become more active to join activities, and share my opinions." (Student D)

> "I used to think that we have to play hard and enjoy everything when we are young. When someone asked me to go out, I would join. But now, I become hardworking. I have something that needs to be fulfilled. I become more aware of my academic performance." (Student E)

Regarding interpersonal competence, the program showed great impacts on building teamwork among the students, enhancing their cooperation with others, and improving their communication skills with others. The paragraphs below highlight some students' sharing on their growth in interpersonal competence:

> "I understand that it is important to cooperate with others. For instance, in the 'university hunt', we needed to find out the answers by ourselves. We were divided into different groups. You could not do it by yourself, and refuse to share with others. You needed to seek help from others. With the limited time, cooperation is very important." (Student F)

"I am a person with very few friends. I always think that two or three friends would be enough for me. But in the 'university hunt', we performed teamwork, and the task was beyond one's capability to be accomplished. And there were more activities that needed cooperation with other persons. I started to realize that I have to open up myself and make more friends. I started to expand my social circle." (Student G)

In addition, Table 3 shows the descriptors used by the students to describe the Project. The students were very positive about the program. Out of 164 descriptors expressed by the students, 160 were positive descriptors (97.6%). The frequently cited descriptors were "amusing," "happy," "exciting" and "interesting," which represented the students' affective responses to the program. At the same time, the students described the program as "practical," "solid" and "meticulous," which illustrated the usefulness and well-organized design of the program. However, a few students found that the duration of the program was too short and the program was too difficult for them. The negative responses (3 out of 164 = 1.8%) were far fewer than the positive responses.

Table 3. Descriptors used by the students to describe the program

Descriptions	Response Positive	Neutral	Negative	Total
Amusing	14			14
Happy	14			14
Interesting	9			9
Practical	8			8
Solid	6			6
Exciting	6			6
Amazing	5			5
Meticulous	5			5
Unforgettable	4			4
Diverse	4			4
Open my eyes	4			4
Inspiring	4			4
Beneficial	3			3
Satisfying	3			3
Gratitude	3			3

Table 3. (Continued)

Descriptions	Positive	Neutral	Negative	Total
Good	3			3
Creative	3			3
Novel	3			3
Enjoyable	3			3
Challenging	3			3
Special	3			3
Enhance confidence	2			2
Caring	2			2
Fantastic	2			2
Meaningful	2			2
Rich content	2			2
Courageous	2			2
Attractive	2			2
Make me hardworking	2			2
Ichiban	1			1
Fast-paced	1			1
Accompanied with me	1			1
Enhance my wellbeing	1			1
Refreshing	1			1
Make me want to try once more	1			1
Relaxing	1			1
Responsive	1			1
Quite good	1			1
Excellent	1			1
Entertaining	1			1
Achieving	1			1
Positive	1			1
Without negative emotions	1			1
Clear	1			1
Friendly	1			1
Responsible	1			1
Educational	1			1
Good timing	1			1
Humorous instructor	1			1
Experiencing	1			1
Wonderful	1			1
Precious	1			1
Cherish	1			1
Understandable	1			1

Descriptions	Response			Total
	Positive	Neutral	Negative	
Touching	1			1
Well-knit	1			1
Long-lasting	1			1
Applicable	1			1
Realistic	1			1
Well planned	1			1
Persistent	1			1
Influential	1			1
No regret	1			1
Difficult to choose		1		1
Short-term			2	2
Difficult			1	1
Total count (N)	160	1	3	164
Total (%)	97.6%	0.6%	1.8%	100%

DISCUSSION

This study examined the perceived benefits of the students after they joined a life and career development program adopting positive youth development approach in Tier 2 Program of Project P.A.T.H.S. In summary, there are several observations of the study. First, analyses of the descriptors of the respondents suggest that the students had very positive responses about the program. Second, aligned with the positive youth development paradigm (8, 9, 12), the life and career development program promoted the psychosocial competence of the students. Regarding intrapersonal development, the program enhanced their self-confidence, courage, resilience and future aspirations. For interpersonal competence, the program strengthened the students' cooperation and communication skills through teamwork. Third, the students had more reflections of their past lifestyles and were motivated to make positive changes. Fourth, the students were more forward-looking in their future paths, and showed eagerness to establish their life goals, formulate their future plans, and research more information on their future aspirations.

Adolescence is the developmental stage when adolescents search for self-identity, independence, intimacy, peer relationships and connections with the outside world (22). It is the time when they develop their competencies so as to make preparation for their transition to adulthood. However, it is also the time when they experience identity confusion, self-doubt, instability and chaos (23, 24). Hence, life and career planning is essential for adolescents to enhance their self-understanding, and formulate their life goals and career development along their life paths. Unfortunately, life and career development programs have been criticized for their narrow scope of information dissemination of educational and vocational opportunities in Hong Kong (25), without taking a wider perspective on the whole-person development. In fact, from the developmental perspectives, life career development is essential for building adolescent self-identity, positive outlook and self-efficacy (6, 26, 27). The present findings also illustrate the effectiveness of the life and career development programs in enhancing the psychosocial development of adolescents, providing strong support for the integration of positive youth development paradigm and life career development model in the adolescent guidance and development programs.

There are several theoretical and practical implications of the study. Theoretically, the integration of positive youth development perspective and life career development is innovative and important to tease out the essential elements of life career development for the adolescents. The findings provide support that adolescents developed their psychosocial competence after participating in the program, and were motivated to pursue their life goals in their future paths. In the rapidly changing and competitive society, adolescents face a lot of challenges that may alter their career choices. Programs merely focusing on vocational development are inadequate and useless (6). What is more important is to develop adolescent competencies and resilience to meet the developmental and ecological challenges. As pointed out by Savickas et al. (28, p. 241),

> "A major consequence of the interconnectedness between the different life domains is that we can no longer speak confidently of

'career development' nor of 'vocational guidance.' Rather, we should envision 'life trajectories' in which individuals progressively design and build their own lives, including their work careers. Not only adolescents will encounter the big question: What am I going to make of my life? This question is at issue for everyone as they negotiate a series of major transitions in their lives occasioned by changes in health, employment, and intimate relationships."

In their views, the importance of positive youth development constructs in determining the essence of life and career development is obvious.

Practically, the participants appreciated the creativity, diversity and usefulness of the program, which gave some threads on the program design of a life and career development program. Rather than using the conventional means of career talks, seminars and exhibitions, teachers and social workers should make use of different program means such as adventure-based training, visits to enterprises and sharing with entrepreneurs, simulation exercises, university visits to arouse adolescents' interest and motivation in their life and career development.

There are several limitations of the study. First, the study was based on the qualitative data collected from focus groups in one secondary school in Hong Kong. There is a need to replicate the study in different schools and community settings. Second, focus group interviews were conducted once at the end of the program. It is recommended to have ongoing evaluation to capture the processes of changes during the intervention. Third, the students were shy and less expressive to share their feelings in a group; more time and encouragement from the moderator would be needed. An alternative is to conduct individual interviews. Fourth, peer checking and member checking were not performed due to the time and manpower constraints, which may reduce the creditability of the study (20). Fifth, more qualitative data collection techniques such as case interviews and reflective journals can help to understand the subjective experiences of the students more deeply.

Despite the limitations, the present study examined the perceived benefits of a life and career development project using the positive youth development approach to enhance the psychosocial development of adolescents in Hong Kong. Essentially, the findings provide important insights for educators, researchers and social workers in the formulation of the future lifelong, holistic, contextual and preventive (28) life and career education in Hong Kong.

ACKNOWLEDGMENTS

The Project P.A.T.H.S. and preparation for this paper were financially supported by The Hong Kong Jockey Club Charities Trust. This paper is based on an article published in the International Journal on Disability and Human Development 2018;17(3) issue. We thank the participants for joining this study.

APPENDIX 1. INTERVIEW GUIDE OF THE FOCUS GROUP

Part 1: Experience of students' participation in the program

- How did you realize this program? How did you enroll in the program?
- What were your expectations before you joined the program? From a retrospective view, how far did the program fulfill your expectations?
- In the program, which part did you like the most? Why?
- In the program, which part did you dislike the most? Why?
- Can you share an occasion/event that you think very impressive? What makes this occasion/event to be the most impressive one? What do you learn from the experience?
- Do you think you are involved in the program? Why or why not?

Part 2: Comments on the program process

- What are your comments on the instructors?
- What are your relationships with the instructors? Do you feel friendly with them?
- Did you know the groupmates before the program?
- Did you have any changes in the relationships with your groupmates? If yes, what are the changes?

Part 3: Comments on the program effectiveness

- What do you benefit the most from the program?
- Did you have any changes after participating in the program? If yes, what are the changes? What makes you have the changes?
- Do you think the program has helped your development? If yes, what are they?
- Do you think the program has helped your adjustment in your school life? If yes, what are they?

Part 4: Overall comments

- Overall, what do you appreciate the most in the program?
- Do you have any suggestions on how the program can be improved?
- If you are invited to use three descriptors to describe the program, what three words will you use?

REFERENCES

[1] Ginzberg E. Toward a theory of occupational choice. Career Dev Q 1988;36(4):358-63.
[2] Super DE. A life-span, life-space approach to career development. In: Brown D, Brooks L, eds. Career choice and development: Applying contemporary theories to practice, 2nd ed. San Francisco, CA: Jossey-Bass, 1990:197-261.
[3] Reardon RC, Lenz JG, Sampson JP, Peterson GW. Career development and planning: A comprehensive approach. Pacific Grove, CA: Brooks/Cole, 2000.
[4] Super DE, Savickas ML, Super CM. The life-span, life-space approach to career development. In: Brown D, Brooks L, eds. Career choice and development: Applying contemporary theories to practice, 3rd ed. San Francisco, CA: Jossey-Bass, 1996:121-70.
[5] Holland JL. Making vocational choices: A theory of vocational personalities and work environments, 2nd ed. Odessa, FL: Psychological Assessment Resources, 1992.
[6] Gysbers NC, Moore EJ. Beyond career development - Life career development. Couns Dev 1975;53(9):647-54.
[7] Gysbers NC, Henderson P. Comprehensive guidance and counseling programs: A rich history and a bright future. Prof Sch Couns 2001;4(4):246-57.
[8] Damon W. What is positive youth development? Ann Am Acad Pol Soc Sci 2004;591(1):13-24.
[9] Shek DTL, Siu AMH, Lee TY. The Chinese Positive Youth Development Scale: A validation study. Res Soc Work Pract 2007;17(3):380-91.
[10] Benson PL. All kids are our kids: What communities must do to raise caring and responsible children and adolescents. San Francisco, CA: Jossey-Bass, 1997.
[11] Lerner JV, Phelps E, Forman Y, Bowers EP. Positive youth development. In: Lerner RM, Steinberg L, eds. Handbook of adolescent psychology, 3rd ed. Hoboken, NJ: John Wiley, 2009:524-58.
[12] Catalano RF, Berglund ML, Ryan JAM, Lonczak HS, Hawkins JD. Positive youth development in the United States: Research findings on evaluation of positive youth development programs. Prev Treat 2002;5(1):Article 15.
[13] Shek DTL, Lee TY. Helping adolescents with greater psychosocial needs: Subjective outcome evaluation based on different cohorts. ScientificWorldJournal 2012;2012:Article ID 694018. DOI: 10.1100/2012/694018
[14] Shek DTL, Sun RCF. Helping adolescents with greater psychosocial needs: Evaluation of a positive youth development program. ScientificWorldJournal 2008;8:575-85.
[15] Lee TY, Shek DTL. Positive youth development programs targeting students with greater psychosocial needs: A replication. ScientificWorldJournal 2010;10:261-72.

[16] Basch CE. Focus group interview: An underutilized research technique for improving theory and practice in health education. Health Educ Behav 1987;14(4):411-48.

[17] Krueger RA. Focus groups: A practical guide for applied research, 2nd ed. Newbury Park, CA: Sage, 1994.

[18] Kitzinger J. Qualitative Research. Introducing focus groups. BMJ 1995;311(7000):299-302.

[19] Shek DTL. The use of focus groups in programme evaluation: Experience based on the Project P.A.T.H.S. in a Chinese context. In: Barbour RS, Morgan DL, eds. A new era in focus group research. Hampshire: Palgrave Macmillan, in press.

[20] Shek DTL, Tang VMY, Han XY. Evaluation of evaluation studies using qualitative research methods in the social work literature (1990-2003): Evidence that constitutes a wake-up call. Res Soc Work Pract 2005;15(3):180-94.

[21] Miles MB, Huberman AM. Qualitative data analysis. Thousand Oaks, CA: Sage, 1994.

[22] Erikson EH. Identity: Youth and crisis. New York: WW Norton, 1968.

[23] Kidwell JS, Dunham RM, Bacho RA, Pastorino E, Portes PR. Adolescent identity exploration: A test of Erikson's theory of transitional crisis. Adolesc 1995;30(120):785-93.

[24] Marcia JE. Identity in adolescence. In: Adelson J, ed. Handbook of adolescent psychology. New York: Wiley, 1980:159-87.

[25] Leung SA. Career counseling in Hong Kong: Meeting the social challenges. Career Dev Q 2002;50(3):237-45.

[26] Bandura A. Adolescent development from an agentic perspective. In: Pajares F, Urdan T, eds. Self-efficacy beliefs of adolescents. Greenwich, CT: Information Age Publishing, 2006:1-43.

[27] Guay F, Senécal C, Gauthier L, Fernet C. Predicting career indecision: A self-determination theory perspective. J Couns Psychol 2003;50(2):165-77.

[28] Savickas ML, Nota L, Rossier J, Dauwalder JP, Duarte ME, Guichard J, et al. Life designing: A paradigm for career construction in the 21st century. J Vocat Behav 2009;75(3):239-50.

In: Psychosocial Needs
Editors: Daniel TL Shek et al.

ISBN: 978-1-53611-951-0
© 2017 Nova Science Publishers, Inc.

Chapter 8

EVALUATION OF A POSITIVE YOUTH DEVELOPMENT PROGRAM FOR LOW-ACHIEVING STUDENTS

Janet TY Leung[1],, PhD and Daniel TL Shek[1-5], PhD, FHKPS, BBS, SBS, JP*

[1]Department of Applied Social Sciences, The Hong Kong Polytechnic University, Hong Kong, PR China, [2]Centre for Innovative Programmes for Adolescents and Families, The Hong Kong Polytechnic University, Hong Kong, PR China, [3]Department of Social Work, East China Normal University, Shanghai, PR China, [4]Kiang Wu Nursing College of Macau, Macau, PR China and [5]Division of Adolescent Medicine, Department of Pediatrics, Kentucky Children's Hospital, University of Kentucky College of Medicine, Lexington, Kentucky, US

In this chapter we present a qualitative evaluation study using focus group methodology to examine the subjective experience and perceived benefits of low-achieving secondary school students who joined the Tier

---

* Correspondence: Janet Leung, PhD, Department of Applied Social Sciences, The Hong Kong Polytechnic University, Hunghom, Hong Kong, PR China. E-mail: janet.leung@polyu.edu.hk.

2 Program of the Project P.A.T.H.S. in Hong Kong. A total of 67 students from eight focus groups participated in the study. Results showed that the students perceived the Tier 2 Program positively as shown by the descriptors they used to describe the Program and the related experience. The students also became more resilient and confident after joining the Program, and many of them showed improvement in teamwork and cooperation with their classmates. The Program enhanced students' relationships with peers, teachers and family members, and they became passionate and motivated to serve the deprived community, especially the elderly. Finally, the students learned to use some constructive ways to resolve conflicts and showed more respect for others. The present study provides evidence on the effectiveness of the positive youth development program in nurturing the holistic development of Chinese adolescents with greater psychosocial needs.

INTRODUCTION

Students' academic underachievement is always linked with problem behaviors. There is empirical evidence that students with poorer academic performance have higher risks of exhibiting internalizing (e.g., depression, anxiety, and withdrawal) and externalizing behavioral outcomes such as delinquency, antisocial behaviors, and bullying in schools (1-3). The effects are amplified when the secondary schools are stratified into different school bands based on the academic standards of the students. With more resources allocated to the schools with more low school achievers, teachers and social workers pay great effort in handling the students' problem behaviors, dealing with their attendance problems, resolving the peer conflicts among students and boosting their academic motivation.

With specific reference to Hong Kong, the present social service orientation is primarily geared towards solving the "problems" of students with low achievement. The "problem" focused orientation generates four fundamental issues. First, it is not effective to remedy the problems and reduce the students' misbehaviors if only remedial measures are offered. There is a common Chinese saying of *"tou tong yi tou, jiao tong yi jiao"* (treat the head when the head aches, treat the foot when the foot hurts) which aptly reflects the limitation of the reactive approach in dealing with adolescent problem behaviors. Second, students are easily labelled as inattentive, misbehaved and problematic, which further lowers their satisfaction with schools and worsens their learning motivation and behaviors (4). Third, teachers and school personnel may need to pay extra effort in resolving teacher-student conflicts that may arise when handling the students' problem behaviors (5), especially when the schools strongly emphasize the enforcement of school regulations and disciplinary practice. Last but not least, the normal developmental needs of the students are ignored. Regardless of their academic performance, adolescents have their normative developmental needs to search for self-identity and recognition by others, build up connections with others and the outside world, and participate in the groups and communities they belong to (6). These are the essential developmental tasks for adolescents to step towards adulthood. Hence, the emphasis of the adolescent problems does not truly respond to the developmental needs of the adolescents.

In recent years, social scientists, educators and social workers have advocated for the use of strengths-based perspective rather than the problem-based perspective in helping needy students (7-9). Saleebey (9) suggested that the strengths perspective is a holistic approach that focuses on the plasticity, resilience and empowerment of an individual in his/her interaction with the environment. Seligman and Csikszentmihalyi (10) explicitly claimed that "our message is to remind our field that psychology is not just the study of pathology, weakness, and damage; it is also the study of strength and virtue. Treatment is not just fixing what is broken; it is nurturing what is best" (p. 7). Shek and Leung (8) also used the analogy of the Western medicine and Chinese medicine to illustrate the importance of building the assets and competencies of an individual in dealing with adversities and challenges. Hence, rather than solely emphasizing the pathology-oriented clinical intervention approach to solve the adolescent behavioral problems, it is more strategic to employ the strengths-based developmental programs to promote competencies and potential of adolescents with greater psychosocial needs.

Table 1. The content of the Tier 2 program

	2013-2014	2014-2015
Adventure-based counseling	• Canoeing	• Canoeing • City Hunt (Tsim Sha Tsui and Central)
Volunteer service	• Home visits to the elderly living in the squatter areas	
Experiential exercises and games	• Class activities	• Class activities • Day camp
Interest learning	• Coffee making • African drum (Djembe)	
Recognition for the students' performance	• Finale cum award presentation ceremony	• Finale cum award presentation ceremony

Against this background, the Project P.A.T.H.S. (Positive Adolescent Training through Holistic Social Programmes) adopting the positive youth development approach was developed to implement a large-scale positive youth development program for junior secondary school students (i.e., Grades 7 to 9) in Hong Kong. There are two tiers in the Project. While the Tier 1 Program makes use of a structural universal curriculum to enhance the interpersonal and intrapersonal competencies of all junior secondary school students, the Tier 2 Program targets the students with greater psychosocial needs and utilizes more diverse intervention strategies and techniques in the program design such as adventure-based counseling, voluntary services, social exposure programs, etc. Undoubtedly, the Tier 2 Program also adheres to the positive youth development paradigm to enhance the positive development of the students.

This chapter examine the effectiveness of a Tier 2 Program delivered to a group of low-achieving students in a secondary school in Hong Kong. The objectives of the Tier 2 Program were: (i) to enhance the psychosocial competencies of the students, and (ii) to increase the exposure of the students. The Program covered eight sessions. Apart from the class activities that aimed at building the cohesion and psychosocial competence of the students, there were different outdoor activities such as day camps, adventure-based counseling programs, volunteer services, and exposure programs, etc. In the Tier 2 Program conducted in 2013-2014, canoeing was organized to build up resilience and courage of the students. Besides, a volunteer service of visiting the single elderly living in the rural areas was designed. Based on the interests of the students, two interest-learning workshops, coffee making and African drum (Djembe), were conducted. Finally, an award presentation ceremony was organized to reward and recognize the efforts and participation of the students.

In the Tier 2 Program held in 2014-2015, a day camp was organized to enhance the team spirit and cohesion among the students. Canoeing was conducted as this activity provided a good platform to develop adolescent resilience and psychosocial competence. Furthermore, a "city-hunt" adventure-based counseling program was organized to enhance the social exposure, persistence, resilience and cooperation among the students. The contents of the Program in each cohort are shown in Table 1. The activities were modified in accordance to the psychosocial needs of the students and recommendations from the school social workers and teachers. In order to make the Program more accessible and attractive, some of the programs were conducted during the school days. Social workers from the non-governmental organization were responsible for conducting the programs and leading the groups. As the Project P.A.T.H.S. was financially supported by The Hong Kong Jockey Club Charities Trust, the programs were free of charge.

This study attempted to examine the effectiveness of a Tier 2 Program delivered to a group of low-achieving students in a secondary school. Two cohorts, 2013-2014 and 2014-2015, of participants were invited to share their views and experiences after joining the Project respectively. A qualitative study of focus group was employed as the research strategy due to four reasons. First, focus group interview effectively taps the perceptions, feelings and opinions of the participants on the programs they involve (11). Second, the group-based format allows the participants to interact with each other and share their experiences together (12). This method is typically welcomed by adolescents as they can communicate with others and share their views in a group. Third, qualitative data would provide rich information for researchers to understand the views and perceptions of the participants, including their subjective experience, the change process, and the rationale behind their choices. Last but not least, many low-achieving students are quite reluctant to fill in the questionnaire due to their constraints of comprehending the statements and questions. Hence, focus group interviews compensate the limitations of using the paper-and-pencil questionnaire.

OUR STUDY

The participants were Secondary 2 students (Grade 8) in a Band 3 secondary school and participated in the Tier 2 Program of the Project P.A.T.H.S. during the academic years of 2013-2014 and 2014-2015. In Hong Kong, the secondary schools are categorized into three bands according to their academic achievements, with Band 3 schools enrolling students having the lowest academic performance. As the selected school belongs to the Band 3 category according to their students' academic performance, many students are "regarded" as low school achievers in the competitive educational ecology in Hong Kong.

In the present study, the students came from one class of Secondary 2 to join the Tier 2 Program of Project P.A.T.H.S. so that more flexibility on the arrangement was allowed. Parental consent to join the Project was sought. There were 33 and 32 students joining the programs in 2013-2014 and 2014-2015 respectively. The selected school was located in the suburban area near the border of China mainland. Some students were immigrants and a high proportion of them experienced economic disadvantage. Sharing the characteristics with many low school achievers, the students were found to have low motivation to study, low self-confidence and poor interpersonal relationships with others.

All students were invited to participate in the focus groups. Informed consent was obtained from both parents and students. Finally, there were 29 and 28 from the two cohorts to join the focus groups respectively. There were a total of eight focus groups conducted for the evaluation within two years.

In each cohort, four focus groups were arranged at the four corners of the school hall. The teachers and school social workers helped to assign the students to different focus groups. There were around five to eight students in each group. The teachers and social workers did not sit in the group so that the students could talk more freely and openly. Each focus group was conducted by a trained researcher who was the moderator of the focus group. The moderator reminded the students to respect one another and adopt an open attitude to accommodate different views and experiences of the participants. Then the moderator conducted the focus group discussion according to an interview guide (see Appendix 1). The students were encouraged to express their views and opinions in the group. The focus group interviews took approximately one hour to complete. All interviews were audio-recorded with the consent of the participants, and the verbatim was transcribed by student helpers from a university.

Though the focus group interview is a useful research strategy to collect the views and opinions of the students, there are two main issues that researchers may need to tackle. First, the interview may be dominant by those students who are more expressive and have stronger views on the Project, making the less expressive students feel hesitant to share their views, especially when their views are different from the so-called "dominant" views. Second, as the students came from the same class, the dynamic relationships among the students may easily influence the atmosphere and participation of the students in the focus group. To avoid the issues, the researchers set some rules and etiquette in the discussion (such as allowing each member to share, showing respect for different opinions, and avoiding rude criticism, etc.). These rules and etiquette may help to build up a more open and friendly atmosphere in the discussion. Besides, the school social workers and teachers helped to arrange the students in different focus groups so as to pace down any undesirable dynamic relationships among the students within each group. As all participants were invited to join the focus groups, no students were excluded from participating in the focus group interviews.

A general qualitative orientation was adopted in this study (13). To interpret the effectiveness of the Tier 2 Program, theme analysis pattern coding was performed. Miles and Huberman (14) suggested that pattern coding is "a way of grouping those summaries into a small number of sets, themes, or constructs ... it's an analogue to the cluster-analytic and factor-analytic devices use in statistical analysis" (p. 69). Principally, the broad themes were extracted from the transcripts of the verbatim. In addition, as the Tier 2 Program aims at enhancing the psychosocial competencies of the students, the perceived benefits were further matched with the 15 positive youth development constructs, namely bonding, resilience, cognitive competence, emotional competence, moral competence, behavioral competence, social competence, spirituality, beliefs in the future, clear and positive identity, self-determination, self-efficacy, prosocial involvement, prosocial norms and recognition for positive behavior (15).

As far as the effectiveness of the Tier 2 Program is concerned, this paper mainly presents the qualitative findings of the comments on the program effectiveness (i.e., Part 3 of the interview guide), as well as the responses of the last question, "If you are invited to use three descriptors to describe the program, what three words will you use?" (Overall comment of Appendix 1). Lastly, the descriptors used by the students to describe the program were categorized into "positive", "neutral" and "negative" responses. This gives us an overview on how the students perceived the Tier 2 Program. The focus group methodology has been used frequently in the project (16).

FINDINGS

Table 2 shows the students' responses on the perceived benefits of the Tier 2 Program. Results showed that students perceived positive changes in both intrapersonal and interpersonal aspects. Regarding the intrapersonal qualities, the students expressed that they became more resilient and confident after joining the programs, especially after participating in the adventure-based counseling programs. The paragraph below highlights a narrative extracted from the focus group with the participants of the Tier 2 Program in 2013-2014:

Moderator: Do you have any changes in the program?
Student A: I think I could get rid of my inferiority, and tried new activities.
Moderator: You have more opportunities to try?
Student A: Yes, my confidence increased.
Moderator: Can you elaborate more?
Student A: I have acquired more knowledge, like the canoeing skills.
Moderator: What do you think the program contributes to your development?
Student A: I have tried out my first step in life, canoeing... I haven't tried this before. I can stand up on the canoe.

Table 2. Students' responses on their perceived benefits of the Tier 2 program

Positive Youth Development Construct	Responses	Frequency	Examples of the Narratives
Resilience	Develop resilience	7	• "(The Program) enhances our life skills when facing adversities. Whenever we face difficulties, we may need to overcome them, and fill up with confidence." • "(The Program) increases my confidence in facing adversities, I have reduced my withdrawal behaviors". • "I have learned the meaning of survival... In case you were in the sea, you must row the boat bravely if you want to survive."
Cognitive competence	Improvement of problem-solving capacity	3	• "I can think of a more gentle problem-solving strategy to solve the problem."
	Build up knowledge and skills	5	• "The Program increases my knowledge, for example, the skills in canoeing."
	Become more conscientious in doing things	2	• "(I) must learn to be very conscientious."
	Be more reflective	3	• "I will do my reflections every night."

Table 2. (Continued)

Positive Youth Development Construct	Responses	Frequency	Examples of the Narratives
Behavioral competence	Build up courage to try new things	5	• "I have the opportunity to try new things that I haven't tried before."
	Learn to reserve resources	2	• "I learn to treasure the resources, and do not make any destructions to things."
	Enhance self-management	2	• "I have to take care of myself. In the past, I used to eat outside and it was expensive. Now I learn to save some money to do something meaningful, such as donation."
	Enhance one's interests	2	• "I learn how to canoe and hope that I can continue to learn more. I hope to reach the fourth star grade."
	Gain new experience and have more life exposure	2	• "I have tried out my first step in life, canoeing…I haven't tried this before. I can stand up on the canoe." • "I have more exposure… (I was) a "villager" (a negative connotation meaning ignorant) before."
Clear and positive identity	Increase self-confidence	9	• "I think I have reduced my inferiority. I tried new things." • "When visiting the elderly, I am more confident to initiate chats with them."
	Become more mature	3	• "What makes the largest difference is that my present feelings and personalities are more mature than in the past. Before that I was like "a frog inside a well" (means ignorant). I did not know anything about the squatter area. But now I visited there and know more about it."
Emotional competence	Have better emotional management	1	• "I have the thought to fight as a way to vent my anger… But now I control myself."
Moral competence	Observe sportsmanship	1	• "(I) learn sportsmanship."
Social competence	Improvement in interpersonal communication skills	10	• "When I chatted with the elderly, I learned the communication skills." • "(I learned) the use of language, and how to respond to others… coming from the experience of talking to the elderly."

Positive Youth Development Construct	Responses	Frequency	Examples of the Narratives
			• "I learned to be open-minded when discussing with others, and felt less shy in communication."
	Build up teamwork	32	• "The Project requires teamwork and how you cooperate with others. Just like in canoeing, when others move forward but you move backward, then we will stay at the original place. You have to cooperate with others." • "(We learn to) cooperate as a team. We have experienced a lot together … as a team, (we face) many challenges and difficulties." • "We have few opportunities to accomplish one task with the whole class. And now we do."
	Show respect for others	3	• "(I) learn how to respect for others…When we have quarrels, I learn how to engage them again."
	Improvement in conflict resolution	3	• "(I) learn how to cooperate with those who have conflicts with me". • "Some people will use violence to resolve (conflicts). We will not use it."
Bonding	Build up companionship	4	• "My relationship with my classmates becomes closer. We interact with each other." • "I have more friends."
	Enhance the bonding with family members	5	• "I treat my family members better…When I visited the elderly and knew that their children did not take care of them, I think when I grow up, I should not neglect my father and mother." • "I learn how to please my grandmother. In the past, I used foul language when I talked to my grandma. But now, I will not." • "It is very helpful for my family. I respect for my grandpa and grandma more, and am polite when talking with them. I learn to value them more. When I visited others (the elderly), they were alone. Therefore, I value them (grandparents) more."

Table 2. (Continued)

Positive Youth Development Construct	Responses	Frequency	Examples of the Narratives
	Improve relationship with teachers and peers in school	4	• "I should respect for the teachers and peers, treasure more people and things around us, and have more interactions with the schoolmates." • "I have better communication with others. Before that, I used to bully on a student, but now I care for him/her."
Prosocial norms	Respect for cultural diversity	3	• "I enjoyed playing African Drum. Others (the players) came from different nations. I learned to respect for them. I was happy with playing with people from other nations." • "I learned not to discriminate against others."
	Respect for the elderly	2	• "The visits to the elderly made me respect for them more."
Prosocial involvement	Become more passionate and motivated to serve others in need	11	• "I learn to care for the poor people in the society. We need to show our concern to them." • "In case I meet someone who are in need, I will help them, for example, giving them some money." • "(We) visited the elderly, made them feel happy. (We) understand more about them, take care of their needs. They will feel our care and concern."
	Understand and show empathy to the elderly	8	• "When I visited the elderly, I found that their lives were really hard. There were many things that they failed to do… buying food, walking downstairs. There were many things that they failed to do… I understood the lives of the elderly more." • "Squatter area…I learned how difficult the lives of the elderly were. There is disparity of the rich and the poor…They have difficulty in buying food." • "When visiting the squatter area, we were exposed to the sunshine, and there were mosquitoes everywhere. You know, the

Positive Youth Development Construct	Responses	Frequency	Examples of the Narratives
			squatters were made of iron, and hence it was very hot inside. The house was hot, and people could not tolerate. The situation is worse in summer when it is 30°C outside, and the house inside would be 40°C. The elderly would have high chance of getting sunstroke...I think the Government is irresponsible. The compensation for the squatter is around $600,000. They could not buy a house with such a small amount of money. They have to wait for the public housing for serval years, and the money would be used up. And they have lived in this area for a long time and have built up affections there. But the Government now wants to redevelop it. The elderly would miss the place very much."

A new and refreshing experience would help the students build up resilience and confidence when they recognized their potential to overcome difficulties. Besides, the students also showed improvement in problem-solving capacities, built up courage to try new things, and became more conscientious, reflective and mature. Some students expressed that they acquired more knowledge, developed new interests, improved emotional management capacities and recognized the importance of sportsmanship. The paragraph below is another narrative of a participant's experience of the Tier 2 Program in 2014-2015:

> Moderator: You've mentioned that you have some improvements. What are they?
> Student B: Ah, on engagement. My teammate had some emotional problems...I wanted to fight with him.
> Moderator: You wanted to fight with him?
> Student B: Yes, fighting, a way to vent my anger.
> Moderator: Oh, and then...
> Student B: I controlled myself.

Regarding the interpersonal competencies, majority of the participants built up their team spirit and enhanced their cooperation with other teammates. They showed more respect for other people and improved their communication skills. It should be highlighted that the students learned how to resolve conflicts when there was disagreement. The paragraph below is a description of the participants joining the Tier 2 Program in 2014-2015:

> *Moderator: What did you learn in the "City Hunt"?*
> *Student C: (I) learned to cooperate with those who had conflicts with me.*
> *Moderator: Before that, how did you treat those people with conflicts?*
> *Student C: We used to quarrel all the time.*
> *Student D: They would fight.*
> *Moderator: How about the most serious quarrel you have ever had?*
> *Student C: The most serious one was that the teacher needed to stop us.*
> *Moderator: But now, how did you interact with them?*
> *Student C: Now, I did not use impolite manner to interact with them... I did not use foul language to talk to them.*
> *Moderator: You are friends now.*
> *Student C: Not really friends, but they are not my enemies.*

Furthermore, the volunteer service in the Tier 2 Program helped to build up the students' passion and motivation to serve the deprived communities, especially the elderly. They understood more on the situations of the elderly and showed empathy for them. In addition, the students' understanding of the needs of the elderly encouraged them to improve the relationship with their parents and care for their grandparents. The paragraph below is a conversation extracted from a focus group on their perceived benefits from the volunteer service in the Tier 2 Program in 2013-2014:

Moderator: Regarding the whole Program, what is the most positive change that you perceive? Can each of you share your view?

Student E: Yes, the visit to a squatter area makes me respect for the elderly more.

Student F: Care for the elderly.

Moderator: From your point of view, do you have any changes?

Student F: When we visited the elderly, I was touched.

Student G: The elderly, I think the Government should pay more attention to the lives of the elderly.

Moderator: But how did this event help or make changes in you?

Student G: I treat my family members better than before.

Moderator: What are the reasons?

Student G: When I visited the elderly and knew that their children did not take care of them, I think when I grow up, I should not neglect my father and mother.

Moderator: Can we say that you have some reflections after the service?

Student G: Yes, probably.

Student H: When I visited the elderly, I found that their lives were really hard. There were many things that they failed to do... buying food, walking downstairs. There were many things that they failed to do.

Moderator: How did this make impacts on you? That is, how did this experience help you? What did you learn?

Student H: I understood the lives of the elderly more.

Moderator: How did this help you?

Student H: I become more caring.

Last but not least, Table 3 shows the descriptors used by the students to describe the Tier 2 Program of the Project P.A.T.H.S. From the feedback of the students, they were positive towards the Tier 2 Program. Out of 79 descriptors used by the students, 72 were positive attributes of the Program. "Amusing", "exciting", "adventurous", "very good" and "interesting" were the most cited descriptors expressed by the students.

Still, some of the students found that the duration of the Project was too short, the Program was not challenging, and a student used the term "suffered" to describe his participation. The negative responses (four out of 79) were far fewer than the positive ones.

Table 3. Descriptors used by the students to describe the Tier 2 program

Descriptions	Positive	Neutral	Negative	Total
Amusing	12			12
Exciting	9			9
Adventurous	7			7
Very good	7			7
Interesting	6			6
Perfect	5			5
Good	3			3
Quite good	3			3
Creative	2			2
New	2			2
Special	2			2
Learn more	2			2
Happy	2			2
Passionate	1			1
Rich content	1			1
Successful	1			1
Hopeful	1			1
Make a difference	1			1
Unique	1			1
Cheap in price	1			1
Challenging	1			1
Funny	1			1
Beautiful	1			1
Average		1		1
Simple		1		1
Easy		1		1
Too short (duration)			1	1
Suffered			1	1
Not challenging			1	1
Hard			1	1
Total count (N)	72	3	4	79
Total Count (%)	**91.14%**	**3.80%**	**5.06%**	**100%**

DISCUSSION

The current study examined the effectiveness of the Tier 2 Program of the Project P.A.T.H.S. from the perspectives of the low achieving students from a secondary school in Hong Kong, with the students divided into eight groups and surveyed in focus group interviews. Several observations can be highlighted in the study. First, the students had positive views of the Tier 2 Program as illustrated by their sharing of the perceived benefits after joining the Program and the descriptors they used to describe the Program. Second, the students expressed that they became more resilient and confident after joining the Program. They also shared some positive changes in the intrapersonal aspects including cognitive competence, emotional competence, behavioral competence and moral competence. Third, a high proportion of the students showed improvement in team building and cooperation with the classmates. Fourth, the Program also enhanced their relationships with peers, teachers and family members. Fifth, the students learned to use some constructive ways to resolve conflicts and showed more respect for other people. Sixth, the students were passionate and motivated to serve the deprived communities, especially the elderly. They were empathetic to the lives of the elderly, which gave them reflections on their relationships with their parents and grandparents, as well as the roles of the government to help the elderly maintain a higher standard of living.

The findings indicated that a higher proportion of the students perceived improvement of teamwork as well as enhancement of resilience and confidence after joining the Tier 2 Program. This is understandable as the adventure-based counseling was emphasized in the program design. The adventure-based counseling program is deliberately used to induce personal growth and development through experiencing and overcoming different challenging tasks (17, 18). Furthermore, both adventure-based counseling and volunteer service required the students to work collaboratively in order to accomplish the tasks (19, 20). Hence, the experiential learning processes through group work enhanced the development of resilience, self-confidence and teamwork.

Several theories account for the associations between adolescent academic achievement and problem behaviors, such as the strain theory (21, 22), the social development model (23) and the problem behavior theory (24). There are also empirical studies showing that low-achieving students were more emotionally vulnerable and exhibited high risks of behavioral problems (25-27). Nonetheless, the potential, passion and competencies of the students should not be ignored. The qualitative findings from the focus groups are strong reminders that though students had low academic achievement, they were passionate to serve the deprived communities in need and strived to achieve when they were encouraged and motivated. At the same time, the students developed their intrapersonal and interpersonal competencies through their involvement and participation. Furthermore, in the review of the poor family socialization theory and deviant affiliation theory that explain the generation of subculture of adolescents in using violence to resolve conflicts and possessing antisocial attitudes towards authority (3, 25, 28), the results are encouraging to reveal that students learned to resolve conflicts positively, observe prosocial norms and improve their relationships with parents and teachers after joining the Tier 2 Program. This provides a strong evidence that positive youth development program serves as a buffer to reduce the detrimental impacts of the negative ecological influences and developmental challenges faced by the adolescents (29, 30).

There are theoretical and practical implications of the study. Theoretically, the study adopted the focus group methodology to examine the perceived benefits of a group of low-achieving students after joining a positive youth development program in Hong Kong. This allows the perceptions of the students to be understood and their voice to be heard. The qualitative findings provide thick descriptions and rich content (31) for the assessment of the effectiveness of a positive youth development program on the adolescents with greater psychosocial needs. More importantly, the study shows the importance on the strengths-based perspective in enhancing the positive development of adolescents with greater psychosocial needs, rather than emphasizing on the deficits, problems and misbehaviors of the low-achieving students. A shift of paradigm on the assessment and intervention of the youth program is worthy to be promoted (8).

Practically, the current study provides evidence that positive youth development program is effective in enhancing the intrapersonal and interpersonal competencies of the low-achieving students. Particularly, the adventure-based counseling programs help to build up resilience, self-confidence and enhance the teamwork of the students. Moreover, the volunteer service is effective in building their passion and prosocial involvement in the society and indirectly improving their relationship with their family members. Hence, adventure-based counseling and service learning approaches are encouraged to be adopted in the positive youth development program for adolescents. These findings are consistent with the previous studies (32-36).

There are several limitations of the study. First, the study was based on the qualitative data of the focus groups in one secondary school in Hong Kong. The school environment may be an influential factor to determine the effectiveness of a positive youth development program for low-achieving students. It is advised to replicate the findings based on participants with similar psychosocial needs in different schools. Second, focus group interviews were conducted at the end of the program at one time point. It is encouraged to have ongoing qualitative evaluation in the study to capture the processes of changes during the intervention. Third, the students may need more time to warm up in the focus group discussion. They did not get used to expressing their feelings and elaborating their ideas publicly in a group. The moderators may need to give more encouragement in the group and adequate time for them to express themselves. Fourth, peer dynamics did influence the focus group discussion. Some students disturbed the discussion frequently. The moderators should be aware of the influence and minimize the disturbance among the students. Fifth, peer checking and member checking were not performed due to the time and manpower constraints, which may reduce the creditability of the study (13). Last but not least, more qualitative evaluation strategies such as in-depth individual interviews are suggested to solicit the subjective experiences of the students.

Despite the limitations, the current study revealed the subjective experiences and perceived benefits of a positive youth development program from a group of low-achieving students in Hong Kong. As Werner and Smith's (37) reminder that "the life stories of the resilient youngsters now grown into adulthood teach us that competence, confidence, and caring can flourish, even under adverse circumstances...From odds successfully overcome springs hope – a gift each of us can share with a child – at home, in the classroom, on the playground, or in the neighborhood" (p. 209), a strengths-based intervention model that nurtures adolescents' competencies and builds their personal assets should be fostered.

ACKNOWLEDGMENTS

The Project P.A.T.H.S. and preparation for this paper were financially supported by The Hong Kong Jockey Club Charities Trust. This paper is based on an article published in the International Journal on Disability and Human Development 2018;17(3) issue. We thank the participants for joining this study.

APPENDIX 1. INTERVIEW GUIDE OF THE FOCUS GROUP

Experience of students' participation in the program
- How did you realize this program? How did you enroll in the program?
- What were your expectations before you joined the program? From a retrospective view, how far did the program fulfill your expectations?
- In the program, which part did you like the most? Why?
- In the program, which part did you dislike the most? Why?

- Can you share an occasion/event that you think very impressive? What makes this occasion/event to be the most impressive one? What do you learn from the experience?
- Do you think you are involved in the program? Why or why not?

Comments on the program process
- What are your comments on the instructors?
- What are your relationships with the instructors? Do you feel friendly with them?
- Did you know the groupmates before the program?
- Did you have any changes in the relationships with your groupmates? If yes, what are the changes?

Comments on the program effectiveness
- What do you benefit the most from the program?
- Did you have any changes after participating in the program? If yes, what are the changes? What makes you have the changes?
- Do you think the program has helped your development? If yes, what are they?
- Do you think the program has helped your adjustment in your school life? If yes, what are they?

Overall comments
- Overall, what do you appreciate the most in the program?

- Do you have any suggestions on how the program can be improved?
- If you are invited to use three descriptors to describe the program, what three words will you use?

REFERENCES

[1] Barriga AQ, Doran JW, Newell SB, Morrison EM, Barbetti V, Robbins BD. Relationships between problem behaviors and academic achievement in adolescents: The unique role of attention problems. J Emot Behav Disord 2002;10(4):233-40.
[2] Hinshaw SP. Externalizing behavior problems and academic underachievement in childhood and adolescence: Causal relationships and underlying mechanisms. Psychol Bull 1992;111(1):127-55.
[3] McEvoy A, Welker R. Antisocial behavior, academic failure, and school climate: A critical review. J Emot Behav Disord 2000;8(3):130-40.
[4] Meilstrup C, Ersbøll AK, Nielsen L, Koushede V, Bendtsen P, Due P, et al. Emotional symptoms among adolescents: Epidemiological analysis of individual-, classroom- and school-level factors. Eur J Public Health 2015;25(4):644-9.
[5] Murray C, Murray KM. Child level correlates of teacher-student relationships: An examination of demographic characteristics, academic orientations, and behavioral orientations. Psychol Sch 2004;41(7):751-62.
[6] Erikson EH. Identity: Youth and crisis. New York: WW Norton, 1968.
[7] Snyder CR, Lopez SJ, Pedrotti JT. Positive psychology: The scientific and practical explorations of human strengths, 2nd ed. Thousand Oaks, CA: Sage, 2015.
[8] Shek DTL, Leung JTY. Adolescent developmental issues in Hong Kong: Phenomena and implications for youth service. In: Shek DTL, Sun RCF, eds. Development and evaluation of positive adolescent training through holistic social programs (P.A.T.H.S.). Heidelberg: Springer, 2013:1-14.
[9] Saleebey D. The strengths perspective in social work practice. Upper Saddle River, NJ: Pearson, 2013.
[10] Seligman ME, Csikszentmihalyi M. Positive psychology: An introduction. Am Psychol 2000;55(1):5-14.
[11] Krueger RA. Focus groups: A practical guide for applied research, 2nd ed. Newbury Park, CA: Sage, 1994.
[12] Kitzinger J. Introducing focus groups. BMJ 1995;311(7000):299-302.
[13] Shek DTL, Tang VMY, Han XY. Evaluation of evaluation studies using qualitative research methods in the social work literature (1990-2003): Evidence that constitutes a wake-up call. Res Soc Work Pract 2005;15(3):180-94.
[14] Miles MB, Huberman AM. Qualitative data analysis. Thousand Oaks, CA: Sage, 1994.
[15] Shek DTL, Siu AMH, Lee TY. The Chinese Positive Youth Development Scale: A validation study. Res Soc Work Pract 2007;17:380-91.
[16] Shek DTL. The use of focus groups in programme evaluation: Experience based on the Project P.A.T.H.S. in a Chinese context. In: Barbour RS, Morgan DL, eds. A new era in focus group research. Hampshire: Palgrave Macmillan, in press.
[17] Ewert A, Yoshino A. The influence of short-term adventure-based experiences on levels of resilience. J Advent Educ Outdoor Learn 2011;11(1):35-50.

[18] Walsh V, Golins GL. The exploration of the outward bound process. Denver, CO: Colorado Outward Bound School, 1976.
[19] Glass JS, Shoffner MF. Adventure-based counseling in schools. Prof Sch Counsel 2001;5(1):42-8.
[20] Leung JTY, Shek DTL. To serve and to learn: Students' reflections of the service learning experience in serving the migrant children in Shanghai. Int J Child Adolesc Health 2016;9(2):165-75.
[21] Cohen AK. Delinquent boys: The culture of the gang. Glencoe, Ill: Free Press, 1955.
[22] Cloward RA, Ohlin LE. Delinquency and opportunity. Glencoe, Ill: Free Press, 1960.
[23] Hawkins JD, Weis JG. The social development model: An integrated approach to delinquency prevention. J Prim Prev 1985;6:73-97.
[24] Jessor R, Jessor SL. Problem behavior and psychosocial development: A longitudinal study of youth. New York: Academic Press, 1977.
[25] Battin-Pearson S, Newcomb MD, Abbott RD, Hill KG, Catalano RF, Hawkins JD. Predictors of early high school dropout: A test of five theories. J Educ Psychol 2000;92(3):568-82.
[26] Bryant AL, Schulenberg JE, O'Malley PM, Bachman JG, Johnston LD. How academic achievement, attitudes, and behaviors relate to the course of substance use during adolescence: A 6 - year, multiwave national longitudinal study. J Res Adolesc 2003;13(3):361-97.
[27] ValÅs H. Students with learning disabilities and low-achieving students: Peer acceptance, loneliness, self-esteem, and depression. Soc Psychol Educ 1999;3(3):173-92.
[28] Hymel S, Comfort C, Schonert-Reichl K, McDougall P. Academic failure and school dropout: The influence of peers. In: Juvonen J, Wentzel KR, eds. Social motivation: Understanding children's school adjustment. New York: Cambridge University Press, 1996:313-45.
[29] Catalano RF, Berglund ML, Ryan JAM, Lonczak HS, Hawkins JD. Positive youth development in the United States: Research findings on evaluation of positive youth development programs. Ann Am Acad Pol Soc Sci 2004;591:98-124.
[30] Sun RCF, Shek DTL. Positive youth development, life satisfaction and problem behavior among Chinese adolescents in Hong Kong: A replication. Soc Indic Res 2012;105(3):541-59.
[31] Leung JTY, Shek DTL. Qualitative and quantitative approaches in the study of poverty and adolescent development: Separation or integration?. Int J Adolesc Med Health 2011;23(2):115-21.
[32] Lee TY, Shek DTL. Positive youth development programs targeting students with greater psychosocial needs: A replication. ScientificWorldJournal 2010;10:261-72.
[33] Shek DTL, Lee TY. Helping adolescents with greater psychosocial needs: Subjective outcome evaluation based on different cohorts. ScientificWorldJournal 2012;2012:Article ID 694018. DOI: 10.1100/2012/694018

[34] Shek DTL, Lee TY, Sun RCF, Lung DWM. Positive youth development programs targeting students with greater psychosocial needs: Subjective outcome evaluation. ScientificWorldJournal 2008;8:73-82.
[35] Shek DTL, Sun RCF. Helping adolescents with greater psychosocial needs: Evaluation of a positive youth development program. ScientificWorldJournal 2008;8:575-85.
[36] Shek DTL, Sun RCF. Evaluation of positive youth development programs that help secondary 2 students with greater psychosocial needs. Int J Public Health 2009;1(3):335-46.
[37] Werner E, Smith R. Overcoming the odds: High-risk children from birth to adulthood. New York: Cornell University Press, 1992.

In: Psychosocial Needs
Editors: Daniel TL Shek et al.

ISBN: 978-1-53611-951-0
© 2017 Nova Science Publishers, Inc.

Chapter 9

DID STUDENTS APPLY WHAT THEY HAD LEARNED FROM A POSITIVE YOUTH DEVELOPMENT PROGRAM IN THEIR REAL-LIFE SITUATIONS?

Tak Yan Lee[*], *PhD, Andrew YT Low, PhD and Anthy LY Ngai*

Department of Applied Social Sciences,
City University of Hong Kong, Hong Kong, PR China

A focus group study was conducted to investigate how adolescent participants perceived and applied the positive youth development (PYD) constructs in their lives during and after joining a two-year PYD program. The longitudinal study attempted to answer two related questions: How effective was the P.A.T.H.S. Project (Phase III) in helping junior secondary school students develop their competencies and skills in terms of PYD constructs? How well did the students apply what they had learned from the program in their real-life situations? Two waves of data

---

[*] Correspondence: Tak Yan Lee, MSW, PhD, Associate Professor, Department of Applied Social Sciences, City University of Hong Kong, Kowloon Tong, Hong Kong, PR China. Email: ty.lee@cityu.edu.hk.

collection with a total of 12 focus group interviews were conducted from six schools with the help of the social workers who carried out the project. In wave 1 data collection, a total of 59 participants from six schools (37 males; 22 females) joined ten focus groups immediately after the completion of the first-year program. Among them, 16 participants from three schools (8 males; 8 females) who completed the second-year program were successfully recruited to join in three focus groups in wave 2 data collection one year after wave 1 data collection. Thematic analysis was used to identify students' recognition and application of PYD constructs in real-life situations. Inter-rater reliability analyses revealed that the coding of students' perceived learning was reliable. From the answers to questions on the experiences gained from the project, most participants perceived the program positively and could give examples related to some PYD constructs to illustrate what they had learned. Selected participants were invited to share concrete examples of application of the PYD constructs after participating in the program. The sharing revealed their development in terms of knowledge, attitude and skills in different PYD constructs.

INTRODUCTION

The Project P.A.T.H.S. (i.e., Positive Adolescent Training through Holistic Social Program, the Project hereafter) which aims at promoting holistic development of adolescents in Hong Kong was first carried out in an Experimental Implementation Phase in 2005/06 (1). In 2006/07, the Full Implementation Phase started on a voluntary basis (2). Phases II and III of the Project were launched from 2009/10 to 2011/12 and from 2013/14 to 2015/16 respectively. As for the program design, the Project used all the 15 positive youth development (PYD) constructs identified by Catalano and his colleagues (3) who reviewed 77 existing PYD programs of which 25 were regarded as successful programs. These 15 positive youth constructs include: a) promotion of bonding, b) promotion of social competence, c) promotion of emotional competence, d) promotion of cognitive competence, e) promotion of behavioral competence, f) promotion of moral competence, g) development of self-efficacy, h) fostering prosocial norms, i) cultivation of resilience, j) cultivation of self-determination, k) promotion of spirituality, l) promotion of beliefs in the future, m) development of clear and positive identity, n) providing opportunities for prosocial involvement and o) providing recognition for positive behavior (3, 4).

Quantitative and qualitative research findings of objective and subjective outcome evaluation (5), process evaluation (6), interim evaluation (2), and randomized controlled trial all showed positive program effectiveness in short-term and long-term reductions in adolescent problem behaviors (7, 8). The Project has received very positive feedback and evaluation results constantly since its inception in 2005. In 2013, the sponsoring body continued to provide funding in supporting the implementation of Phase III of the Project, titled "Community-based Youth Enhancement Program". No participating schools in this phase had joined the Project formerly. In Phase III, the same design was used – primary prevention in the format of a universal program named as Tier 1 program for all students in Secondary 1 to 3 (S1 to S3) together with a secondary prevention program (Tier 2) targeting students with greater psychosocial needs. Tier 2 program activities were designed by the school social work agency with reference to the 15 PYD constructs as well as the needs of the participants. The dominant approaches were adventure-based activities as well as volunteer training and service (9).

Extensive research was done to investigate the effectiveness of the Project in Phases I and II (10-12). The results showed positive feedback from the majority of respondents regarding the program contents, effectiveness and quality of the program. In Phase III, initial research focused on subjective outcome evaluation by the program implementers and program participants, resulting in generally positive feedback and successful program implementation (13-15). However, previous evaluations focused mainly on the program contents, perceived program effectiveness in terms of positive development, short-term (7) and long-term reductions in adolescent problem behaviors (8), willingness of recommendation of the program to others and satisfaction with the program. Therefore, this study is concerned with the participants' perceived learning and application of the PYD constructs in the real-life situations. While many studies had been conducted to illustrate the outcomes in terms of the desirable and undesirable behaviors, the mediating role of PYD constructs has not been examined.

This is the first study which adopted the qualitative approach to study the effects of the Project P.A.T.H.S. through interpreting participants' real-life experiences using the PYD constructs. Adopting the thematic approach to examine the concrete examples given by the participants, we were able to identify how participants perceived their learning in the program and how they applied what they had learned to their daily lives to show the effects of the program from the participants' perspective.

Two objectives were addressed in this longitudinal qualitative research. First, the research specifically examined the effectiveness of the PYD program in promoting PYD constructs. Second, this research focused on participants' learning and applications of the PYD constructs by examining their real-life experiences within the first two years of the program implementation period.

OUR STUDY

There were 174 schools joining Phase III of the Project P.A.T.H.S. in 2013, involving a total of 5,042 students. The Project was carried out in two tiers providing primary and secondary prevention services respectively. Tier 1 is a universal and primary prevention program for all students and Tier 2 program serves students who have greater psychosocial needs identified by parents, teachers, and/or through self-report questionnaires (16). After careful selection of participants, Tier 2 program serves as the secondary prevention program. According to the social workers who provided services to the participating schools, psychosocial needs of participants in this research included but not limit to those having difficulties in school adjustment, inadequate social skills as well as low self-efficacy and self-esteem. Among all Tier 1 program participants, 2,754 were Secondary 1 students, 888 were students from Secondary 2 and 1,400 were students from Secondary 3. About one-fifth of Secondary 1 and Secondary 2 students were selected to join the Tier 2 program.

The sampling process involved inviting two different social welfare agencies providing school social work service for six schools. One of the agencies provided services to two schools and another agency served four schools. In total, 74 students were invited from these six schools to participate in the focus group interviews. They were all Tier 2 program participants. Given the nature of the longitudinal research, two waves of data collection were conducted. The first one was conducted immediately after the first-year program was completed. These 74 participants were invited to join the focus group interview again after the second-year program. In wave 1, a total of eight focus group interviews with 58 Secondary 1 students from six schools were conducted during February to June 2014. However, three schools dropped out in wave 2 data collection. Therefore, only three focus group interviews with 16 Secondary 2 students from three schools were organized between May and July, 2015. Table 1 shows the demographic data of the interviewees. Although the attrition rate was very high (i.e., 72.8%), the number of participants joining the two waves of data collection was acceptable due to the nature of a qualitative study.

Table 1. Demographic information of the interviewees from six schools

School code	Wave 1			School code	Wave 2		
	Total numbers	Male	Female		Total numbers	Male	Female
A (Group 1): A1	5	0	5	A3 (Wave 2)	6	0	6
A (Group 2): A2	7	0	7		6	0	6
B (Group 1): B1	8	8	0	B3 (Wave 2)	5	5	0
B (Group 2): B2	12	12	0		5	5	0
C (C1: Wave 1)	7	4	3	C2 (Wave 2)	5	3	2
D	7	4	3	*	nil	nil	nil
E	6	5	1	*	nil	nil	nil
F	7	4	3	*	nil	nil	nil

Note: * Three schools withdrew from wave 2 data collection

One agency which served two schools arranged written parental consent because the interviews took place outside of the school premises. Another agency did not arrange written parental consent as the interviews were conducted during the normal school hours. Participants were invited to take part in the focus group interviews by the school social workers. Verbal explanations on the purposes, procedures and privacy protection measures were given to the potential participants. The researchers also obtained verbal consent from the interviewees before the interviews started.

Two researchers with social work training conducted the focus group interviews jointly, facilitating participants to verbalize their perceptions, learning from the program, and their application experiences. With consent from the participants, the process of interviews was audio-taped. Participants were encouraged to express their opinions after joining the program. The same interview guide was used in the two waves of interviews. Table 2 shows the interview questions of the focus group interviews.

Table 2. Interview questions of the focus group interviews related to positive youth development constructs with program participants

General Impression of the Program
Do you have any unforgettable experiences about your participation in this program?
Evaluation of the Effectiveness of the Program
Do you think that the program has helped your development?
After participating in the program, do you have any changes? If yes, please specify. (free elicitation)
What have you gained in this program? (free elicitation)
Do you think the program can enhance your abilities in different areas in your life?
What are the most useful things that you learned during the process? Can you provide some examples?

Inter-rater reliability was used to ascertain the reliability of coding. After the two waves of interviews, two research assistants selected lines that potentially reflected PYD constructs and coded each line independently. After initial coding, research assistants counted the frequency of the different constructs. The correlation coefficients between the frequencies of constructs identified by the two coders are calculated. The inter-rater reliability is the correlation coefficients. In general, the correlation coefficient of coding between the two raters is high, except one of which the reliability of all the other ten groups were above 0.74 ($p < 0.05$). Table 3 shows the reliability of the coding of the PYD constructs between the two raters for the different focus group interview sessions.

Table 3. Reliability of the coding of the PYD constructs between the two raters for different focus group interview sessions

School code	Wave 1 Reliability	Overall	School code	Wave 2 Reliability	Overall
A1	.647**	.806***	A3	.911**	.83**
A2	.744**				
B1	.784**		B3	.833**	
B2	.756**				
C1	.739**		C2	.742**	
D	.75**		*	nil	nil
E	.876**		*	nil	nil
F	.81**		*	nil	nil

Note: * Three schools withdrew from wave 2 data collection.
The inter-rater reliability is the correlation coefficients between the frequencies of constructs identified by the two coders. ** $p < 0.05$. *** $p < 0.01$.

Thematic analysis was employed to analyze the data obtained from the focus group interviews. Thematic analysis is a qualitative research method for "identifying, analyzing and reporting themes within data" (17) (p. 79). The phases of thematic analysis developed by Braun and Clarke (17) are adopted in data analysis. In the first step of familiarizing with the data, the research assistants transcribed the recorded dialogues and another research staff checked the accuracy of the transcription. In the second step of generating the initial codes, the research assistants marked the responses that might show the relevance of the PYD constructs. Additionally, in order to enhance triangulation of coding, a total of three researchers read and marked the ideas for coding independently. In the third step of searching for themes, the research assistants coded the selected responses in terms of the PYD constructs and also took notes of the difficulties in coding. Reference to the definitions of each PYD construct was based on the literature. In the fourth step of reviewing the themes, the identified constructs were reviewed independently by two researchers in order to determine the most representable construct for each selected response. The data obtained after coding were analyzed using the frequency counts. The final step of "naming and defining themes" was omitted because the coding was based on the 15 PYD constructs. Finally, the verbatim illustrating how some participants used what they had learned from the program activities was cited.

WHAT WE FOUND

All 15 PYD constructs were found. Table 4 shows the frequency counts of the constructs by the two independent raters in waves 1 and 2 respectively. The constructs that were not found by any rater in any of the focus group interviews were excluded from further discussion. As a result, eight constructs with the highest percentage of appearance based on the total frequency counts of both waves of data collection were identified. They are: a) social competence (24.36%), b) prosocial involvement (13.69%), c) emotional competence (10.19%), d) resilience (9.39%), e) prosocial norms (7.25%), e) self-efficacy (6.39%), g) behavioral competence (6.21%), and h) bonding (4.62%). Since prosocial involvement and prosocial norms were closely related, these two constructs were grouped together as a single theme. Generally speaking, students showed improvements and learning in these eight constructs.

Table 4. Frequency counts of the PYD constructs coded by the two raters

Constructs	Wave 1 Data Rater A Frequency	Rater A %	Wave 1 Data Rater B Frequency	Rater B %	Wave 2 Data Rater A Frequency	Rater A %	Wave 2 Data Rater B Frequency	Rater B %	Total (Frequency)
Social Competence (SC)	52	33.77	54	30.17	28	15.56	19	16.52	153 (24.4%)
Prosocial Involvement (PI)	45	29.22	20	11.17	8	4.44	13	11.30	86 (13.7%)
Emotional Competence (EC)	8	5.19	18	10.06	24	13.33	14	12.17	64 (10.2%)
Resilience (RE)	4	2.60	23	12.85	22	12.22	10	8.70	59 (9.4%)
Prosocial Norms (PN)	12	7.79	9	5.03	14	7.78	10	8.70	45 (7.3%)
Self-Efficacy (SE)	9	5.84	12	6.70	11	6.11	8	6.96	40 (6.4%)
Behavioral Competence (BC)	3	1.95	3	1.68	22	12.22	11	9.57	39 (6.2%)
Bonding (BO)	6	3.90	6	3.35	9	5.00	8	6.96	29 (4.6%)
Cognitive Competence (CC)	0	0.00	4	2.23	14	7.78	7	6.09	25 (4%)
Spirituality (SP)	10	6.49	10	5.59	0	0.00	0	0.00	20 (3.2%)

Table 4. (Continued)

Constructs	Wave 1 Data						Wave 2 Data						Total
	Rater A			Rater B			Rater A			Rater B			(Frequency)
	Frequency	%		Frequency	%		Frequency	%		Frequency	%		
Self-Determination (SD)	3	1.95		0	0.00		11	6.11		8	6.96		22 (3.5%)
Clear and Positive Identity (ID)	1	0.65		11	6.15		3	1.67		1	0.87		16 (2.6%)
Recognition for Positive Behavior (RB)	0	0.00		9	5.03		2	1.11		1	0.87		12 (1.9%)
Moral Competence (MC)	1	0.65		0	0.00		9	5.00		0	0.00		10 (1.6%)
Beliefs in the Future (BF)	0	0.00		0	0.00		3	1.67		5	4.35		8 (1.3%)
Total	154	100%		179	100%		180	100%		115	100%		628 (100%)
Reliability		0.806*						0.83*					

Note: The inter-rater reliability is the correlation coefficients between the frequencies of constructs identified by the two coders, *$p < 0.05$.

All schools organized volunteer training and services (VTS) and adventure-based activities (ABAs) for the participants in the Tier 2 program. The choice of activities might influence participants' perceived impacts of the program. The findings of this study are generally consistent with the previous studies, showing positive program effectiveness from students' perception. The seven themes identified in the present study further demonstrate participants' understanding and conscious application of the PYD constructs in their real-life situations. Concrete examples will be presented after a brief discussion.

Improvement in social competence

Social competence refers to three important aspects, including a) ability of interpersonal conflicts resolution and development of positive and healthy interpersonal relationship; b) development of clear self-identity, and a group or collective identity; and c) the orientation of being responsible and caring citizens locally and globally (18, 19). Literature on social competence emphasizes the development of the interpersonal relationship and the concept of identity which consists of personal, group, social, and national identities necessary for the development of citizenship (18, 19).

> "After joining the program, I realized that I had great improvements personally. In primary school, I liked playing games and mobile phone at home at weekends. After the program, I reduced my reliance on my mobile phone, computer or television. It's because I began to understand human relationship is the most important thing. Although you could use your phone or computer, you may not have better communication than face-to-face communication." (C1_225)
>
> "You need to understand other people's perspectives, for example, why he shouted at me or what my stance is…I need to consider the stance of both sides." (D_533)
>
> "For example, if we could understand each other more, we could learn to be considerate, which would then reduce the chance of bullying." (D_542)

"In the past, we might complain easily, but now we are more considerate and show concern for our friends." (B1_460)

"For example, setting up a fire for barbecue... if we do it alone without other people's help, we cannot make it. If there is someone to help, we can do it together and realize that it is not difficult." (E_120)

Some participants used their real-life examples to illustrate improvements in their interpersonal relationship. They developed their group identities through the program which successfully cultivated the positive interpersonal relationship among the participants. This then helped them develop prosocial behavior (20). Given that the program helped the students establish the positive interpersonal relationship and increase their abilities to resolve the interpersonal conflicts, it is likely that the program could enhance the participants' self-identity and citizenship.

Increased prosocial involvement and reinforced prosocial norms

Prosocial norms and prosocial involvement are two closely related but different PYD constructs. Prosocial involvement refers to activities with the purpose of benefiting others (21). Prosocial norms refer to behavioral guidelines, unambiguous, healthy, ethical standards, beliefs, and beliefs that minimize health hazards and promote prosocial behavior (22). Mazur (23) stated that responsibility, reciprocity, volunteerism and altruism are the common prosocial norms that youth development programs promote.

Successful cultivation of prosocial norms was observed through participation in the adventurous tasks and voluntary service which required cooperation, mutual help, sharing and communication as well as learning how to care about the elderly and the visually impaired. Specifically, some participants expressed that the activities had increased their understanding of the disadvantaged groups in society. The following examples of changes in behavior and attitudes correspond to the current literature about ability of empathy and its positive connection to prosocial behavior (21, 24).

"In this program, we had chances to connect with the community. For example, we could understand the needs and thoughts of the elderly after visiting the elderly home." (B3_110)

"My family does not have any old people so I do not know how to get along with the elderly. After we visited the elderly home, I learned to get along with them, such as using the appropriate words." (C2_39)

"For people who did not help as a volunteer in the past, this program could provide opportunities for them to be a volunteer and learn how to take care of the elderly." (B3_119)

Furthermore, students had more empathetic understanding of the lives and difficulties of the visually impaired people. Therefore, they showed more acceptance and consideration to people with visual impairment. Some participants expressed that they are willing to offer help to the needy in the real-life situations.

"The social worker organized an event about the visually impaired people. The activity was to simulate how the visually impaired people walk. Our eyes were covered by a blindfold and we were led by another student. I realized that it was a very difficult situation. For example, it is very inconvenient and easy to get hurt. I felt that it is very unfortunate to be a person with disability. I started to show concern for others and tolerate others even when they do something wrong. I become less stubborn." (C2_43)

"I learned to avoid laughing at and making fun of others. I learned to be considerate toward others." (C1_49)

"When I see people who are blind, I will try to help them." (C2_54)

The program provided the chances of prosocial involvement and further encouraged the participants to adopt clear, positive, healthy, and ethical standards in planning and joining the prosocial activities. Some participants showed empathetic understanding of the elderly's and the visually impaired people's needs and characteristics. They were able to transform their experience from the voluntary service to the real-life situations (21). Additionally, some participants improved their communication skills when they got along with the elderly.

Improvement in emotional competence

Emotional competence is a strong predictor of life success and is especially important in youth development (25). Lau (26) stated that the operational definition of emotional competence consists of three components, including skills for a) identifying personal feelings and those of others, b) communicating emotions with others, and c) coping with negative emotions and difficult situation. Some participants revealed behavioral changes when they were invited to talk about emotional competence after joining the program. Compared with their behavior before joining the program, a participant identified improvement in the awareness of his/her own emotions and discerning others' emotions in wave 2.

"When we were climbing a rope, some people were responsible for pulling the rope. Communication is needed between one another. It was because I would hit the wall if they pulled too tight or too loose. Therefore, I learned to communicate with people. If people do not like listening, I would talk less, listen to them first, and to add my opinions later." (A3_57).

Additionally, some participants expressed that they learned skills about communication of emotions and expression of feelings. They acknowledged the importance to communicate feelings and thoughts instead of suppressing emotions.

"After joining the program, I became braver to express my own opinions. In the past, I would let people talk first. I was timid. Now I prefer to express my opinions. I see that other shy students are also brave enough to express their opinions now. Therefore, I learn from them and express my own thoughts bravely." (F_174 & F_176)

Furthermore, some participants perceived themselves as having better skills to cope with the negative emotions. They acknowledged the importance of emotional management and tendency of reducing self-harm behavior. They became more patient when dealing with the interpersonal relationships by applying the skills learned from the training session on emotion and temperament management.

> "I know from the news reports, many teenagers have self-harm behavior nowadays. I heard that some students in my school did that but it was anonymous. The social worker explained to us about the experience of the suicidal incidents. We learned how to control our emotions better. There is no need to hurt ourselves. It is better to talk to a social worker or do something else instead of self-harming." (C_544)
>
> "When I have conflicts with my siblings, I am more tolerant now. I would not lose my temper and give them a punch. Although we argue, I would now show my tolerance instead of cursing immediately as I was before." (A3_178)

The above examples illustrate that some participants were able to utilize different strategies to express their emotions, show their empathy and sympathy for others' emotional experiences, realize the differences between their own emotional states and outer emotional expression, cope with the negative emotions in a proper way, and understand the importance of reciprocal sharing to build an intimate relationship with others (26).

Enhancement of resilience

Resilience is a multidimensional construct which encompasses components of capacity, process and result. It is defined as a process of using internal and external resources effectively in order to adapt or manage significant stress or trauma (27). Promotion of resilience refers to fostering capacity and flexibility as well as using coping strategies when facing life stresses and developmental changes so as to "bounce back" from adversity in life and attain positive outcomes (8, 28, 29). Smith (30) summarized both internal and external protective factors for resilience. Internal protective factors include optimism, perceptions of control, and self-efficacy. External protective factors include bonding, competence (i.e., cognitive, emotional, behavioral and social competence), optimism, and a supportive environment.

> "Rope climbing can cultivate perseverance in ourselves. It helps us be braver, able to face challenges... and we would not withdraw." (F_290)
>
> "It seems that I have built more self-confidence in social activities." (A2_1014)
>
> "In the program, I was so scared to join the night walk because of the darkness and the possibility of getting lost. I reached the destination in the end. In the past, I would have just ignored things that I did not know how to do. I might try doing other stuff first. Now, I think of other possible solutions. If I cannot think of any alternatives, I would seek help from others." (A3_99)
>
> "The process of serving others also contributes to identifying my strengths, potential, and passions, which finally leads to a clearer identity." (B2_120)

Resilience involves the interaction of other PYD constructs, for example, bonding, self-efficacy, cognitive competence, emotional competence, behavioral competence and social competence (27). To illustrate the enhancement of resilience, the participants' perceived capacity, coping strategies and flexibility in facing difficulties are shown. Some participants revealed that they learned to be more capable in facing difficulties and became more flexible in solving problems during the program. Furthermore, some participants used the real-life examples to illustrate that they were able to apply what they learned to analyze the situations, make workable decisions and be optimistic when they faced adversities (31).

Enhanced self-efficacy

To accomplish developmental tasks, children need to accumulate experiences. Self-efficacy beliefs play an important role in attributing the lack of success to inadequacies in skills or knowledge, maintaining perseverance in completing a task, keeping an intrinsic interest in the work and life tasks, having the vision to treat difficulties as opportunities for development, sustaining the desire to attain more demanding goals, and recovering quickly after failure (32). Some participants were able to identify behavior and performance in activities and tasks taken in the program and attribute the success to their psycho-social-moral functioning.

"I was afraid of darkness in the past. I became braver after the night walk. I was able to get up in the dark and turn on the light on my own." (A1_321)

"We had to plan and prepare games for the elderly. After that event, I could think of many interesting things easily." (B2_442)

"We (Secondary 2) served as leaders to help Secondary 1 students provide the voluntary services for the elderly. S1 students were young and they did not know much. We had to keep telling them what to do and what not to do. We were able to carry out the service and were very happy because the elderly were very happy." (C2_31)

"In the past, I was indecisive and unable to make immediate decisions. Last summer, I went hiking. The guide asked us to turn left in a road junction. We followed the instruction but we walked to a dead end. Therefore, we had to make a decision of what to do. If I didn't make a prompt decision, it would be too dark to carry on. However, we were not familiar with the mountain area and the district was not well developed. Therefore, it was dangerous. We had to make an immediate decision. I made a quick decision to walk back to the original road. We were able to get out of the mountain. I felt thankful that I could make a prompt decision." (D_107)

The above illustrations show that some participants' self-efficacy beliefs were enhanced through successful completion of the adventurous tasks and voluntary service. The sense of mastery, the use of vicarious experiences and persuasion, which require cognitive, motivational, affective abilities, are demonstrated.

Improvement in behavioral competence

Ma (20) defined behavioral competence by four parameters including a) moral and social knowledge: learning social-moral values, social norms, laws, and regulations in groups, such as home and school; b) social skills: the ability to behave socially, morally desirable in daily interaction with other people by using non-verbal and verbal strategies; c) positive characters and attributes: the development of positive characters and prosocial orientation; and d) behavioral decision process and action taking: the process of making behavioral decision and taking action to carry out the decision. Promotion of behavioral competence in early adolescence requires the availability of assistance to develop skills to perform normative behaviors such as apology, criticism, applause, refusal, and help to enable them to make effective behavioral choices and take actions through verbal and non-verbal communication (20, 33).

"After I visited the social service agency for people with visual impairment, I met one of the members of the agency when I took the train. I saw that he had to get off the train in a station but no one offered help to him. Therefore, I accompanied him from the platform to the exit. However, I cannot help him further because I had to take a transit for my violin class. If I did not join these activities, would I be indifferent to people with visual impairment? Would I choose to help him if I did not visit the agency? I think the program helped me (to understand the needy and to help them)." (C1_58)

"In primary school, I had many conflicts with my friends. I would ignore them or grin and bear it. However, I would reflect what I did wrong now and apologize for it." (A3_93)

"Some people are strong-minded and consider their opinions as the most important. It seems that their views are absolutely correct. They simply ignore opinions of others and refuse to change their mind. After joining this program, I realized that and started to reflect if I had similar weakness too. I begin to ask others for opinions and see if I have to improve in some areas." (C1_147)

"In this activity, I think that adolescents can learn how to be considerate toward others. We either win or lose in a game. For the losing group, it is common that the failure is caused by a member who does not take the game seriously. Similarly, in the activities of this program, some groups lost the game because of the fault made by an individual group member. Despite that, we learned to tolerate and forgive the wrongdoing of that groupmate and we became more considerate toward others. At first, some members blamed others for losing the game. In the end, we understood that we needed teamwork indeed. So we should have team spirit. From time to time, students knew how to express themselves when they lost the game. For example, 'Never mind!', 'Don't care about the results.', and 'The most important thing is to enjoy the process'." (C1_149)

Apart from the social skills required in the construct of social competence, some participants stressed that they had significant improvement in moral and social knowledge as well as the development of positive characters and attributes. It was observed that students gained moral and social knowledge and developed positive characters. For instance, students reflected that they were willing to take the responsibility for their wrongdoing. In short, some were able to behave with prosocial motivation. The program activities facilitated the development of socially acceptable normative behavior, characters and manners. However, improvements in decision-making process and action taking were not widely identified.

Enhanced bonding with family members

Bonding is defined as a person's emotional attachment and commitment to social relationships with parents, caregivers, peers, schoolmates, siblings, teachers, romantic partners, and other individuals of the community throughout one's life cycle (28, 34-39). Particularly, bonding to parents and school are protective factors moderating the developmental risks of adolescents (3, 40).

"I cared more for the elderly. I know how to take care of them." (B1_419 & B1_422)

"I learned to care for others. I learned to treasure friendship and I love my parents." (B2_240 & B2_243)

"We need to be considerate toward the elderly because their hearing is deteriorating. We need to repeat what we've said and stop complaining about their long-winded behavior." (A1_100)

"After visiting the elderly home, I really felt that I need to spend more time with my grandmother." (A3_979)

Some participants acknowledged their development of a strong affective relationship with their parents and peers in the school. When the participants were invited to talk about their experience in volunteer training and voluntary services, they revealed having an improved communication with their family members. Additionally, some participants noted that they became more compassionate and concerned with their family members, especially the older generation.

Limitations and future research

The present study has several limitations. First, the sample size in wave 1 was 59 and was only 16 in wave 2. The attrition rate was as high as 72.8%. Moreover, all interviewees were recruited by the school social workers who organized the PYD program. Sample bias could not be ruled out. The sampling issue dampens the generalizability and validity of the results. Second, the interviewees with stronger verbal abilities appeared to tell more concrete examples of applying the PYD constructs while those with weaker verbal abilities seemed not to be able to tell examples in detail even with repeated encouragement. Perhaps the group size should be further reduced so that more time could be provided for the less vocal participants to speak in the focus groups. Third, the Chinese cultural context of Hong Kong may affect substantially the results and therefore makes them specific to Hong Kong. Some characteristics such as filial obedience, filial piety, collectivism, and humbleness may facilitate the PYD program to achieve its effectiveness (41). Fourth, the schools offered different extracurricular activities for their students at the same time when the program was implemented. The PYD program participants might have difficulties in differentiating clearly the effects of the program and those attributable to other extracurricular activities. They might have learned knowledge and skills from other channels that were also helpful to their psycho-social-moral development. When the interviewees were asked for examples of applying what they learned from the program, they might not be able to distinguish the learning from various sources. Even though the participants were asked to recall the particular activities unique to the program before they gave application examples, it is conceivable that the interviewees might have applied what they learned from other sources. Therefore, a causal relationship between the PYD program and the participants' successful application of PYD constructs in real-life settings cannot be ascertained. Fifth, the program implementers are excluded from data collection and analysis. The absence of data triangulation threatens the validity of the study. Moreover, to avoid over-interpretation and misinterpretation of the data, the present study focused discussion on the constructs with higher frequency counts. Although some constructs, for example, beliefs in future and spirituality were mentioned in the focus group interviews, it limited the possibilities to understand if students gained insights in these constructs. Finally, due to the time and manpower constraints, the research participants were not involved in choosing or agreeing with the themes and conclusion drawn. To provide a more complete study on the effectiveness of the program, Carey (42) suggested that opinions of the participants can be used to justify the choice of themes and the related conclusion.

Future research can build on the present study by clarifying the contributions of specific program activities according to the theory of change. Processes of change can then be transparent in future research.

ACKNOWLEDGMENTS

The preparation for this paper and the Project P.A.T.H.S. were financially supported by The Hong Kong Jockey Club Charities Trust. This paper is based on an article published in the International Journal on Disability and Human Development 2018;17(3) issue. We thank the participants for joining this study.

REFERENCES

[1] Shek DTL, Sun RCF. Implementation of the Tier 1 Program of the Project P.A.T.H.S.: Interim Evaluation Findings. ScientificWorldJournal 2006;6:2274-84.
[2] Shek DTL, Ma HK, Sun RCF. Interim evaluation of the Tier 1 Program (Secondary 1 Curriculum) of the Project P.A.T.H.S.: First year of the full implementation phase. ScientificWorldJournal 2008;8:47-60.
[3] Catalano RF, Berglund ML, Ryan JAM, Lonczak HS, Hawkins JD. Positive youth development in the United States: Research findings on evaluations of positive youth development programs. Prev Treat 2002;5(1):Article 15. DOI: 10.1037/1522-3736.5.1.515a.
[4] Cheng HCH, Siu AMH, Leung MCM. Recognition for positive behavior as a positive youth development construct: Conceptual bases and implications for curriculum development. Int J Adolesc Med Health 2006;18(3):467-73.
[5] Shek DTL. Effectiveness of the Tier 1 Program of the Project P.A.T.H.S.: Preliminary objective and subjective outcome evaluation findings. ScientificWorldJournal 2006;6:1466-74. DOI: 10.1100/tsw.2006.238.
[6] Shek DTL, Ma HK, Lui JH, Lung DW. Process evaluation of the Tier 1 program of the Project P.A.T.H.S. ScientificWorldJournal 2006;6:2264-73.
[7] Shek DTL, Siu AMH, Lee TY, Cheung CK, Chung R. Effectiveness of the Tier 1 program of Project P.A.T.H.S.: Objective outcome evaluation based on a randomized group trial. ScientificWorldJournal 2008;8:4-12. DOI: 10.1100/tsw.2008.16.
[8] Catalano RF, Fagan AA, Gavin LE, Greenberg MT, Irwin Jr CE, Ross DA, Shek DTL. Worldwide application of prevention science in adolescent health. Lancet 2012;379(9826):1653-64.
[9] Lee TY, Shek DTL. Positive youth development programs targeting students with greater psychosocial needs: A replication. ScientificWorldJournal 2010;10:261-72. DOI: 10.1100/tsw.2010.3.

[10] Shek DTL, Lee TY, Sun RCF. Evaluation of a youth development program in the Experimental Implementation Phase. Int J Adolesc Med Health 2008;1(2):169-82.

[11] Shek DTL. Using student weekly diary to evaluate positive youth development programs: The case of Project P.A.T.H.S. in Hong Kong. Adolescence 2009;44(173):69-85.

[12] Shek DTL, Sun RCF. Qualitative evaluation of the Project P.A.T.H.S. (Secondary 1 Program) based on the perceptions of the program implementers. Int Public Health J 2009;1(3):255-66.

[13] Shek DTL, Ma CMS, Xie Q. Evaluation of a community-based positive youth development program based on Chinese junior school students in Hong Kong. Int J Adolesc Med Health 2016. Epub ahead of print 14 Jun 2016. DOI: 10.1515/ijamh-2017-3002.

[14] Shek DTL, Ng CSM, Law MYM. Community-based positive youth development program in Hong Kong: Views of the program Implementers. Int J Adolesc Med Health 2016. Epub ahead of print 14 Jun 2016. DOI: 10.1515/ijamh-2017-3003.

[15] Shek DTL, Ng CSM, Law MYM. Positive youth development programs for adolescents with greater psychosocial needs: Evaluation based on program implementers. Int J Adolesc Med Health 2016. Epub ahead of print 14 Jun 2016. DOI: 10.1515/ijamh-2017-3005.

[16] Shek DTL, Ma HK. Design of a positive youth development program in Hong Kong. Int J Adolesc Med Health 2006;18(3):315-28.

[17] Braun V, Clarke V. Using thematic analysis in psychology. Qual Res Psychol 2006;3(2):77-101.

[18] Ma HK. Social competence as a positive youth development construct: Conceptual bases and implications for curriculum development. Int J Adolesc Med Health 2006;18(3):379-85.

[19] Ma HK. Social competence as a positive youth development construct: A conceptual review. ScientificWorldJournal 2012;2012:Article ID 287472. DOI: 10.1100/2012/287472.

[20] Ma HK. Behavioral Competence as a positive youth development construct: A conceptual review. In: Shek DTL, Sun RCF, Merrick J, eds. Positive youth development: Theory, research, and application. New York: Nova Science, 2013:189-200.

[21] Lam CM. Prosocial Involvement as a positive youth development construct: A conceptual review. ScientificWorldJournal 2012;2012:Article ID 769158. DOI: 10.1100/2012/769158.

[22] Eisenberg N, Carlo G, Murphy B, Court P. Prosocial development in late adolescence: A longitudinal study. Child Dev 1995;66(4):1179-97.

[23] Mazur JE. Learning and behavior, 2nd ed. Englewood Cliffs, NJ: Prentice-Hall, 1990.

[24] Fabes RA, Carlo G, Kupanoff K, Laible D. Early adolescence and prosocial/moral behavior I: The role of individual processes. J Early Adolesc 1999;19(1):5-16.

[25] Wang N, Young T, Wilhite SC, Marczyk G. Assessing students' emotional competence in higher education: Development and validation of the Widener Emotional Learning Scale. J Psychoeduc Assess 2010;29(1):47-62.

[26] Lau PS. Emotional competence as a positive youth development construct: Conceptual bases and implications for curriculum development. Int J Adolesc Med Health 2006;18(3):355-62.

[27] Lee TY, Cheung CK, Kwong WM. Resilience as a positive youth development construct: A conceptual review. ScientificWorldJournal 2012;2012:Article ID 390450. DOI: 10.1100/2012/390450.

[28] Choi PYW, Au CK, Tang CW, Shum SM, Tang SY, Choi FM, Lee TC. Making young tumblers: A manual of promoting resilience in schools and families. Hong Kong: Breakthrough, 2003. [Chinese].

[29] Wong KY, Lee TY. Professional discourse among social workers working with at-risk adolescents in Hong Kong: Risk or resilience? In: Ungar M, ed. Handbook for working with children and youth: Pathways to resilience across cultures and contexts. Thousand Oaks, CA: Sage, 2005:313-27.

[30] Smith BW. Vulnerability and resilience as predictors of pain and affect in women with arthritis. Doctoral dissertation. Tempe: Arizona State University, 2002.

[31] Gillham J, Reivich K. Cultivating optimism in childhood and adolescence. Ann Am Acad Pol Soc Sci 2004;591(1):146-63.

[32] Tsang SKM, Hui EKP, Law BCM. Self-efficacy as a positive youth development construct: A conceptual review. ScientificWorldJournal 2012;2012:Article ID 452327. DOI: 10.1100/2012/452327.

[33] Ma HK. Behavioral competence as a positive youth development construct: Conceptual bases and implications for curriculum development. Int J Adolesc Med Health 2006;18(3):387-92.

[34] Ainsworth MDS. Attachments and other affectional bonds across the life cycle. In: Parkes CM, Stevenson-Hinde J, Marris P, eds. Attachment across the life cycle. London: Tavistock/Routledge, 1991:33-51.

[35] Berndt TJ. Friendship quality and social development. Curr Dir Psychol Sci 2002;11(1):7-10.

[36] Fisher CB, Lerner RM, eds. Encyclopedia of applied developmental science. Thousand Oaks, CA: Sage, 2005.

[37] Klaus MH, Kennell JH, Klaus PH. Bonding: Building the foundations of secure attachment and independence. Reading, MA: Addison-Wesley, 1995.

[38] Lee TY, Lok DPP. Bonding as a positive youth development construct: A conceptual review. ScientificWorldJournal 2012;2012:Article ID 481471. DOI: 10.1100/2012/481471.

[39] Wilks J. The relative importance of parents and friends in adolescent decision making. J Youth Adolesc 1986;15(4):323-34.

[40] Catalano RF, Oesterle S, Fleming CB, Hawkins JD. The importance of bonding to school for healthy development: Findings from the social development research group. J Sch Health 2004;74(7):252-61.
[41] Lee TY, Shek DTL, Kwong WM. Chinese approaches to understanding and building resilience in at-risk populations. Child Adolesc Psychiatr Clin N Am 2007;16(2):377-92.
[42] Carey M, ed. Qualitative research skills for social work: Theory and practice. Aldershot: Ashgate, 2012.

In: Psychosocial Needs
Editors: Daniel TL Shek et al.

ISBN: 978-1-53611-951-0
© 2017 Nova Science Publishers, Inc.

Chapter 10

DOES STUDENTS' ACADEMIC ABILITY MAKE A DIFFERENCE IN THE LEARNING OUTCOMES OF A POSITIVE YOUTH DEVELOPMENT PROGRAM IN HONG KONG?

Tak Yan Lee*, PhD, Andrew YT Low, PhD, Jerf Yeung, PhD and Yuki X Jin
Department of Applied Social Sciences,
City University of Hong Kong, Hong Kong, PR China

In this chapter we attempt to examine the effectiveness of the Project P.A.T.H.S., a positive youth development (PYD) program, among a specific sample of secondary students in Hong Kong, taking into consideration for the context of academic ability grouping. The sample consists of 59 Secondary 1 students from six schools. For the evaluation of their developmental outcomes, eight focus group interviews were conducted to collect data. Interviews were conducted in their schools with the help of school social workers. Content analysis was employed to

---

* Correspondence: Tak Yan Lee, MSW, PhD, Associate Professor, Department of Applied Social Sciences, City University of Hong Kong, Kowloon Tong, Hong Kong, PR China. Email: ty.lee@cityu.edu.hk.

examine the project participants' perceived effectiveness of the program according to the experiential learning theory (1). Cohen's kappa statistic was used to check inter-judgmental agreement between two raters on the frequencies of five components of experiential learning. Statistics showed that there is very high agreement ($k > 0.80$) in the coding of experiential learning processes of participants. Separate Chi-square analyses showed significant relationships between academic ability grouping and abstract conceptualization ($p < 0.01$), action taken ($p = 0.011$), but not reflective observation or planning for action, an extra construct used in this study. The results, according to the developmental outcomes of this sample, have allowed us to identify the most significant impact related to the academic ability grouping and consider its implications for future program design and implementation.

INTRODUCTION

Phase 3 of the Project P.A.T.H.S. is named Community-based Positive Youth Development (PYD) program with an aim to reach out to schools that have not yet participated in the program. With the same aim to promote holistic youth development and quality of life as in the previous phases, the project extended its coverage to more adolescents in Hong Kong. The program has two distinct tiers. Tier 1 provides universal coverage for all Secondary 1 students through classroom learning with specially designed curriculum units (2) while Tier 2 program targets at students with greater psychosocial needs. By using adventure-based activities (ABAs) and volunteer training and service (VTS), Tier 2 program aimed to foster participants' interest and engagement in activities, and to promote broader psychosocial, emotional, and behavioral development. For a PYD program aiming to help all students in Hong Kong, we are interested in understanding whether participants with different academic ability levels would have differential learning outcomes. Through a qualitative outcome evaluation, this study examines how the Project P.A.T.H.S. benefited participants, with the purpose to identify critical design features to maximize positive outcomes through a large PYD program.

Academic ability grouping in Hong Kong

Before entering into secondary schools, students in Hong Kong are classified into three equally sized bands within each school district according to their levels of academic ability/achievement in primary schools. To distinguish the differences in schools' internal assessment, students sit through low-stake achievement tests in Chinese, Mathematics and English towards the end of the primary school. The purpose of the tests is to ensure a fair comparison of internal results of schools and the mechanism is designed to reduce the stress arising from high-stake tests. Instead of assessing the merit of individual students, the schools' overall results are scaled. Students will then fall into three bands. In allocating primary students to secondary schools, students with the highest ability/achievement levels can be allocated to Band 1 while those with the lowest level are placed in Band 3 (3). Students of the same banding are assigned to government or aided schools (4). While teachers of Band 1 students can use English as the medium of instruction (MOI), teachers of Band 3 students use their mother tongue (Cantonese) as the MOI. For Band 2 students, teachers may use English supplemented by Cantonese or using English textbooks in order to enhance students' English language ability as far as possible.

The mechanism of allocation of secondary school places based on banding has been practiced in Hong Kong for many years. Homogeneous group of students based on ability/achievement could allow teachers to use different MOI to maximize educational results (5). Moreover, Lou and colleagues (6) found that students could cooperate better, experience mutual facilitation, and learn at the same pace.

What could possibly be the relationship between students' academic ability grouping and their learning through the PYD program? Will students of different bands gain different outcomes in the Project P.A.T.H.S.? To answer these questions is the major purpose of this study.

Experiential learning

For the evaluation of learning outcomes, Kolb (1) argues that learning should focus on the process of learning as opposed to the behavioral outcomes. His theory, named as experiential learning theory (ELT) distinguishes experiential learning from the idealistic approaches of traditional education and from the behavioral theories. Kolb contends that learning is a continuous process characterized by four stages, i.e., Concrete Experience (CE), Reflective Observation (RO), Abstract Conceptualization (AC) and Active Experimentation (AE) (1, 7-9).

Considering participants were mostly 11 to 13 years old, they were helped by school social workers in the process of the Tier 2 program, receiving training in volunteer service, and engaging in planning and carrying out a visit, usually an elderly home to provide service. We have further differentiated active experimentation (AE) into planning for action (AE1) and action taken (AE2) respectively.

Given that there is no research on the relationship between students' banding and PYD outcomes, and having in mind that banding has been the widely accepted standard in the Hong Kong education system, this paper aims at examining the experiences of participants of the Project P.A.T.H.S. from two different bands, i.e., Band 1 and Band 3, and to find if there are any differences. The results could inform professionals in the process of providing secondary prevention programs for students with greater psychosocial needs. Therefore, our aim is to examine the effectiveness of the Phase 3 of the Project P.A.T.H.S, with a focus on exploring whether banding will make a difference in the Tier 2 program. It is hypothesized that participants from different bands would yield statistically different results in terms of PYD outcomes through the Tier 2 program process. i.e., CE, RO, AC, AE1, and AE2.

OUR STUDY

Fifty-nine Secondary 1 students were invited from six schools to participate in the focus group interview. They were participants of the

Phase 3 of Project P.A.T.H.S.. All participants were ethnic Chinese. There were 37 (62.7%) boys and 22 (37.3%) girls in the convenience sample. School social workers invited participants to join the interview. Among all participants, 31 were Band 1 students from two schools using English as the medium of instruction (EMI) while 28 were Band 3 from four schools where the medium of instruction is Chinese (CMI). Table 1 shows the demographic data of interviewees.

For the students from two Band 1 schools, written informed consents were obtained from their parents because the interviews were arranged to take place outside of school premises immediately after an after-examination activity. Informed verbal consents were also obtained before the focus group interview through the help of the school social workers. For those Band 3 students recruited from four schools, only informed verbal consents were obtained through the help of the school social workers because the interviews took place at the schools. Verbal explanations on the purposes, procedures and privacy protection measures were given to potential participants. Two researchers with social work training conducted the focus group interview jointly. Participants were encouraged to express their opinions after joining the program, including but not limited to learning that specifically related to the positive youth development constructs. Table 2 shows the interview guide of the focus group interviews. With informed consent from participants, the process of interviews was audio-taped.

Table 1. Demographic data of interviewees

School	Group Code	Number of participants	Male	Female
A	A1	5	0	5
	A2	7	0	7
B	B1	8	8	0
	B2	12	12	0
C	C1	7	4	3
D	D	7	4	3
E	E	6	5	1
F	F	7	4	3
	Total	59	37	22

Table 2. Interview guide for the focus group interviews with program participants

General Impression of the Program
Do you have any unforgettable experiences concerning your participation in this program?
Evaluation of the Effectiveness of the Program
Do you think that the program has helped your development?
After participating in the program, do you have any changes? If yes, please specify (free elicitation).
What have you gained in this program? (free elicitation)
Do you think the program can enhance your abilities in different areas in your life?
What are the most useful things that you learnt during the process? Can you provide some examples?

Kolb's experiential learning cycle (1) was employed and slightly modified to measure students' intention and actual participation in certain activities that were related to PYD. The cycle starts with an encounter of new experience (Concrete Experience, CE). For example, participants joined a night walk, a camp, a volunteer training or service in the Tier 2 program. The second stage is reflective observation (RO), in which adolescents have a break from "doing" thus allowing them to step back from the task and review what they have done and experienced in relation to past experience and conceptual understandings. Abstract conceptualization (AC) refers to the process of making sense of what have happened, and involves in interpreting the events as well as figuring out the relationships between them, such as giving theories, concepts or present models that may clarify implications for an action. Active experimentation (AE) is the last stage of Kolb's experiential learning cycle (9). However, we distinguish two levels of AE in our study. When the learners consider how they can adopt what they have learnt in practice, we define it as planning for action (AE1) and when they have already applied what they learned in the world around, this experience is defined as action taken (AE2). So the final step of the learning cycle is completed.

The focus group interviews were audio-recorded and the verbatim was transcribed into texts in the format of verbatim lines with school and line code added in the database. Two raters reviewed and rated each line from the five dimensions (CE, RO, AC, AE1, and AE2) as 'high or a lot' (i.e., value = 1) or 'low or no' (i.e., value = 0).

Content analysis is an approach to summarize any form of contents by counting various aspects of the contents. Underlying meanings and ideas can be revealed by analyzing patterns in the texts, including words or phrases (10). In this study, texts are empirically coded according to a researcher's created coding system in order to "make observation about the messages conveyed" (11, p. 286). This allows a more objective evaluation than simply summarizing contents based on the impressions of a listener.

Cohen's kappa statistic (k) is a measure of chance-corrected reliability of ratings, and was used to determine inter-rater reliability in developmental outcomes between participants with varying academic performance. The maximum possible k is 1 (100%), indicating perfect inter-judgmental agreement. A value of 0 indicates that agreement is entirely attributable to chance. The degree of inter-judgmental concordance is described as: poor (<0.20); fair (0.21-0.40); moderate (0.41-0.60); substantial (0.61-0.80); and almost perfect (0.81-1.00) (12).

Pearson's Chi-square analyses were also employed to evaluate how well the observed distribution of coded "data fits with the distribution that is expected if the variables are independent" (13, p. 594).

Separate chi-square tests were adopted to examine the differences between the two groups of participants (i.e., Band 1 (EM1) and Band 3 (CMI)) along the five dimensions. This allows us to test the hypotheses of differences.

OUR FINDINGS

Based on the agreement on modified rating scheme of the experiential learning process, two examiners finished their ratings independently. Overall, almost perfect agreement was obtained at all calculations

(*Kappa* >0.80). Viewed in this context, the coding of the learning process in terms of PYD outcome is highly reliable. Table 3 presents the kappa coefficients in the two groups along five dimensions.

Table 3. Cohen's Kappa statistics for agreement between two raters on the five learning stages by two groups of participants

	Learning Stages	Cohen's Kappa
Band 1: EMI	CE	1
	RO	0.967
	AC	0.811
	AE1	0.855
	AE2	0.964
Band 3: CMI	CE	1
	RO	1
	AC	0.954
	AE1	0.772
	AE2	0.948

Table 4. Chi-square Test on Academic ability grouping and Learning Outcomes

Variable Name		df	*p value*	Significance
RO	Reflective observation	1	0.478	
AC	Abstract conceptualization	1	<0.01	<0.01
AE1	Planning for action	1	0.841	
AE2	Action taken	1	0.011	<0.05

The results revealed no significant relationship between academic ability grouping and reflective observation (RO) or planning for action (AE1) (See Table 4). However, significant differences were found between academic ability grouping and abstract conceptualization (AC) (92.9% as compared to 66.7%, see Table 5) ($p < 0.001$), as well as action taken (AE2) (33.3% as compared to 16.7%, see Table 6) ($p = 0.011$). Tables 4 to 6 detail the statistics.

Table 5. Frequency distribution of Abstract Conceptualization (AC) by Banding

			Band One	Band Three	Total
AC	No	Count	9	14	23
		% within Band	7.1%	33.3%	13.6%
	Yes	Count	118	28	146
		% within Band	92.9%	66.7%	86.4%
Total		Count	127	42	169
		% within Band	100.0%	100.0%	100.0%

Table 6. Frequency distribution of Action Taken (AE2) by Banding

			Band One	Band Three	Total
AE2	No	Count	84	60	144
		% within Band	66.7%	83.3%	72.7%
	Yes	Count	42	12	54
		% within Band	33.3%	16.7%	27.3%
Total		Count	126	72	198
		% within Band	100.0%	100.0%	100.0%

DISCUSSION

This paper extended the current literature on the outcome evaluation of PYD by taking academic ability grouping into consideration. These findings suggest that students from different levels of academic performance (banding) did not reveal any differences in their exposure to new experience, reflective observation or planning for new behavior with regard to experiential learning through the Tier 2 PYD program. Both Band 1 and Band 3 students could clearly recall their concrete experiences during the adventure-based activities, including night walk, camping, as well as volunteer training and service. They could express what they learned from such activities. Consistent with findings from previous evaluation studies of the project P.A.T.H.S., over 80% of all program participants opined that the program improved their competencies at the societal, familial, interpersonal and personal levels and their quality of life (14-16).

However, it is found that these two groups displayed differences in the frequencies of coded abstract conceptualization (AC) and actual action of applying learned experience into daily life (AE2). Especially, Band 1 students seem to benefit more than their Band 3 counterparts in these two aspects. As expected, Band 1 students revealed great capacity to conceptualize (17) and to act (18). It is conceivable that Band 1 students — who presumably possess better understanding in abstract knowledge and finer skills in knowledge transfer — also gained faster and deeper understanding of the meaning of the PYD program activities that they had joined. Besides, higher levels of behavioral self-regulation were associated with higher academic skills (18). That might explain why the two groups revealed similar intention to act, yet significant differences in whether they performed or not. Given that both groups of participants have gone through similar program activities, the question of how to promote deeper understanding (AC) of the experiences and encourage more actual experimentation in terms of actual application of what they learn in real life situation among Band 3 students is raised. This could be one of the future research questions.

Another plausible explanation is that the socio-economic status may contribute to the differences (19). Band 1 students may have more resources (3). They may come from more affluent families which allow easier access to diverse educational and developmental resources (20, 21).

Moreover, academic ability grouping allows students with similar ability level to be assigned to the same school. Peer influence and cooperation reinforce mutual learning among them. Further studies may focus on the peer culture and the school social worker's role in helping students from different academic ability grouping in order to maximize program effectiveness.

Furthermore, Band 1 students may be more responsive and active in class (22, 23). At the same time, they were also more active in response to questions raised by the interviewers.

On the contrary, Band 3 students may experience difficulties in academic during their primary school years due to having less educational and familial resources. They may have lower self-esteem and hesitate to verbalize their feelings, thoughts and experiences in the group interview out of the fear of rejection and criticism (24). However, it is possible that interviewers might need more time in building a good rapport with the interviewees in the focus groups, making it easier to engage Band 3 students to verbalize the program effects. This is one of the major limitations of this study. Follow up qualitative studies with program participants are needed to rule out the possible effect of limitation in verbal expression of their learning experiences.

Contrary to our hypothesis, no significant differences were observed between the two groups in reflective observation and planning for action. In terms of reflective observation, it is possible that the memory of the experiences in the Project P.A.T.H.S. is equally fresh to both groups since the interviews were conducted within one month following the completion of the Tier 2 program. In this sense, we do not know if the differences are still non-significant after some period of time. The retention of program effects can be examined to further study the difference between the two groups by adopting a longitudinal research design. Positive intention responses show that both groups have good planning skills. This could probably be the effective work of the school social workers in the Tier 2 program.

To conclude, this study provides pioneering qualitative research findings on the learning stages of Band 1 and Band 3 students participating in the Tier 2 PYD programs of the Project P.A.T.H.S.. The present study differentiates two related and yet different components of the last stage of Kolb's experiential learning theory (1), i.e., planning for action (AE1) and actual action of applying learned experience into daily life (AE2). The results suggest that Band 1 students seem to benefit more than their counterparts of Band 3 in two of the five different stages of the experiential learning theory - abstract conceptualization (AC) and actual action (AE2). Statistically significant differences were found in these two aspects. Consistent with the literature, Band 1 students revealed great capacity to conceptualize (17) and to act (18). However, the cohort study design could not rule out the possibility that Band 1 students are more capable to describe their learning experience gained from the PYD program activities through the use of abstract terms.

Since the Project P.A.T.H.S. is designed for all students, the research question on whether there is any difference in the learning outcomes among students with varying academic ability levels is important. The findings of this study have important implications for future program design and implementation particularly for PYD program implementers working with Band 3 students. It is suggested that more effort and skills in interaction and debriefing (25-29) are needed to help students with lower academic or language ability.

Acknowledgments

The preparation for this paper and the Project P.A.T.H.S. were financially supported by The Hong Kong Jockey Club Charities Trust. This paper is based on an article published in the International Journal on Disability and Human Development 2018;17(3) issue. We thank the participants for joining this study.

References

[1] Kolb DA. Experiential learning: Experience as the source of learning and development. Upper Saddle River, NJ: FT press, 2014.
[2] Shek DTL. Effectiveness of the tier 1 program of the Project P.A.T.H.S.: Preliminary objective and subjective outcome evaluation findings. Scientific WorldJournal 2006;6:1466-74.

[3] Salili F, Lai MK. Learning and motivation of Chinese students in Hong Kong: A longitudinal study of contextual influences on students' achievement orientation and performance. Psychol Schools 2003;40(1):51-70.

[4] Chong CSC, Forlin CI, Au ML. The influence of an inclusive education course on attitude change of pre - service secondary teachers in Hong Kong. Asia - Pac J Teach Educ 2007;35(2):161-79.

[5] Rudowicz E, Hui A. School banding and creativity of Hong Kong junior secondary school students. Educ Res J 2002;17(1):43-62.

[6] Lou Y, Abrami PC, Spence JC. Effects of within-class grouping on student achievement: An exploratory model. J Educ Res 2000;94:101-12.

[7] Kolb DA, Fry RE. Toward an applied theory of experiential learning. Cambridge, MA: MIT Alfred P Sloan School Management, 1974.

[8] Kolb DA. Experiential learning: experience as the source of learning and development. Englewood Cliffs, NJ: Prentice-Hall, 1984.

[9] Kolb AY, Kolb DA. Experiential learning theory. In: Seel NM, ed. Encyclopedia of the sciences of learning. Boston, MA: Springer, 2012:1215-9.

[10] Yang K, Miller GJ. Handbook of research methods in public administration, 2nd ed. Boca Raton, FL: CRC Press, 2008.

[11] Babbie ER. The basics of social research, 8th ed. Belmont: Wadsworth, 1999.

[12] Viera AJ, Garrett JM. Understanding interobserver agreement: The kappa statistic. Fam Med 2005;37(5):360-3.

[13] Gravetter FJ, Wallnau LB. Statistics for the behavioral sciences. Belmont, CA: Wadsworth Cengage Learning, 2013.

[14] Shek DTL, Ma CMS, Xie Q. Evaluation of a community-based positive youth development program based on Chinese junior school students in Hong Kong. Int J Adolesc Med Health 2016. Epub ahead of print 14 Jun 2016. DOI: 10.1515/ijamh-2017-3002.

[15] Shek DTL, Ng CSM, Law MYM. Community-based positive youth development program in Hong Kong: Views of the program implementers. Int J Adolesc Med Health 2016. Epub ahead of print 14 Jun 2016. DOI: 10.1515/ijamh-2017-3003.

[16] Shek DTL, Law MYM. Evaluation of programs for adolescents with greater psychosocial needs: Community-based Project P.A.T.H.S. in Hong Kong. Int J Adolesc Med Health 2016. Epub ahead of print 14 Jun 2016. DOI: 10.1515/ijamh-2017-3004.

[17] Cacioppo JT, Petty RE, Kao CF. The efficient assessment of need for cognition. J Pers Assess 1984;48:306-7.

[18] von Suchodoletz A, Gestsdottir S, Wanless SB, McClelland MM, Birgisdottir F, Gunzenhauser C, et al. Behavioral self-regulation and relations to emergent academic skills among children in Germany and Iceland. Early Child Res Q 2013;28(1):62-73.

[19] Sirin SR. Socioeconomic status and academic achievement: A meta-analytic review of research. Rev Educ Res 2005;75(3):417-53.

[20] Chiu MM, Ho ESC. Family effects on student achievement in Hong Kong. Asia Pac J Educ 2006;26(1):21-35.
[21] Chiu MM, Walker A. Leadership for social justice in Hong Kong schools: Addressing mechanisms of inequality. J Educ Admin 2007;45(6):724-39.
[22] Lounsbury JW, Sundstrom E, Loveland JM, Gibson LW. Intelligence, "Big Five" personality traits, and work drive as predictors of course grade. Pers Indiv Differ 2003;35(6), 1231-9. DOI:10.1016/S0191-8869(02)00330-6
[23] Vermetten YJ, Lodewijks HG, Vermunt JD. The role of personality traits and goal orientations in strategy use. Contemp Educ Psychol 2001;26(2):149-70.
[24] Wong MSW, Watkins D. Self-esteem and ability grouping: A Hong Kong investigation of the big fish little pond effect. Educ Psychol 2001;21(1):79-87.
[25] Fagan AA, Mihalic S. Strategies for enhancing the adoption of school-based prevention programs: Lessons learned from the blueprints for violence prevention replications of the life skills training program. J Commun Psychol 2003;31(3):235-53.
[26] Ennett ST, Ringwalt CL, Thorne J, Rohrbach LA, Vincus A, Simons-Rudolph A, et al. A comparison of current practice in school-based substance use prevention programs with meta-analysis findings. Prev Sci 2003;4(1):1-14.
[27] Shek DTL, Sun RCF. Implementation of a positive youth development program in a Chinese context: The role of policy, program, people, process, and place. ScientificWorldJournal 2008;8:980-96.
[28] Shek DTL, Sun RCF. Implementation quality of a positive youth development program: Cross-case analyses based on seven cases in Hong Kong. ScientificWorldJournal 2008;8:1075-87.
[29] Shek DTL, Sun RCF. Development, implementation and evaluation of a holistic positive youth development program: Project P.A.T.H.S. in Hong Kong. Int J Disabil Hum Dev 2009;8(2):107-18.

In: Psychosocial Needs
Editors: Daniel TL Shek et al.
ISBN: 978-1-53611-951-0
© 2017 Nova Science Publishers, Inc.

Chapter 11

THE EXPERIENCES OF EARLY ADOLESCENTS AFTER JOINING A POSITIVE YOUTH DEVELOPMENT PROGRAM

Andrew YT Low[*]*, PhD, Tak Yan Lee, PhD and Roger KL Lau*
Department of Applied Social Sciences,
City University of Hong Kong, Hong Kong, PR China

The present chapter attempts to ascertain the effectiveness of a positive youth development (PYD) program through qualitative interview of the program participants to understand their perception about the program by asking them to recall their subjective perception of the results of the intervention. Two waves of qualitative data were collected immediately after the completion of the program and one year after the program respectively. A total of eight groups of early adolescents aged 12 to 14 who successfully completed the program attended semi-structured interviews. The results indicated retention in some but not all impacts one year after the completion of the program. Furthermore, participants

---

[*] Correspondence: Andrew YT Low, PhD, Assistant Professor, Department of Applied Social Sciences, City University of Hong Kong, Kowloon, Hong Kong, PR China. Email: yiutlow@cityu.edu.hk.

opined that they were satisfied with life, established and had a higher level of self-discipline.

INTRODUCTION

The purpose of this chapter is to present and analyze the findings of an evaluation of the phase III of Project P.A.T.H.S. (Positive Adolescent Training through Holistic Social Programs, the Program hereafter). It is a program which aims to facilitate adolescent holistic development in Hong Kong. It is a universal program premised on positive developmental constructs proposed by Catalano and his colleagues (1). The 15 positive youth development constructs include spirituality, prosocial norms, prosocial involvement, beliefs in the future, clear and positive identity, self-efficacy, self-determination, moral competence, behavioral competence, cognitive competence, emotional competence, recognition for positive behavior, social competence, resilience, and bonding (1). The experimental implementation phase (phase I) was carried out in the 2005/06 school year, which was followed by the full implementation phase in 2006/07. From 2009/10 to 2012/13, P.A.T.H.S. phase II was successfully implemented. The program's effectiveness has been depicted by different qualitative and quantitative studies, which include the subjective and objective outcome evaluation findings (2), longitudinal objective outcome evaluation (3, 4), interim evaluation (5), qualitative evaluation (6) and case studies (7). In view of the success, The Hong Kong Jockey Club Charities Trust has provided funding to support the continuation of the Project P.A.T.H.S, giving birth to phase III in 2013/14.

A longitudinal study was adopted by this research to remedy the lack of evaluation of youth development projects over a period of time (8). Replication over time is an important element in the realm of science (9). Adopting the growth curve modeling (IGC) approach, previous longitudinal research has supported the claim that Project P.A.T.H.S. has long-term effects in adolescent problem prevention (7, 10), especially in the promotion of the positive development of young people (8). The longitudinal studies on the Project P.A.T.H.S. have been focusing on quantitative measures of the 15 constructs identified by Catalano and his colleagues (1), and a composite measure on the positive youth development scale. Previous qualitative studies focused on participants' perspective on what they had learnt. This study has expanded the realm of previous research by evaluating the program's effectiveness through quantitative content analysis. Different perceived impacts were coded based on the dialogs of participants without referring to the 15 constructs. Students' personal insight on their learning was recorded and coded. The current study offers a more comprehensive view on the longitudinal effect of the Project P.A.T.H.S.

Theoretical framework

The present phase of the Project P.A.T.H.S. is composed of program activities aiming to enhance positive development of adolescents identified as having greater psycho-social needs (11). The program activities include adventurous activities, voluntary services and emotional management groups. The adventurous activities include night walks, team-building activities and problem-solving activities. In the voluntary services, participants need to learn to plan and deliver an activity to serve the needy in the community. Examples include visits to the elderly homes, centers for people with physical disabilities, and child-care centers.

Adventure-based activities

Adventure-based counseling (ABC) constitutes a mix of group counseling, experiential learning, outdoor activities and intrapersonal exploration, which utilize some levels of risk to achieve therapeutic changes (12). The adventure-based activity (ABA) is one of the essential elements in ABC. ABA itself facilitates therapeutic changes such as enhancing the wellbeing of young people and helping them to feel calmer, happier, more positive and optimistic (13). In addition, young people are more able to manage risky situations after joining ABC. ABA also enhances group cohesion, increases the sense of cooperation among young people and also reduce fear and anxiety in their lives. Fletcher & Hinkle (12) indicated that ABC is based on the behavioral and cognitive theories. It also constitutes the concept of experiential learning. This is a form of counseling that facilitates learning by doing. It has been identified that ABC is able to promote personal growth, accountability, support and trust among participants. Studies also indicate an enhancement in self-concept and the sense of well-being of participants after joining the program (13). Another important theoretical concept is the "comfort zone model," which serves as the basis on which a majority of adventure education practitioners deliver the ABC. This model suggests that participants in a stressful or challenging situation will respond to and cope with the occasion. After overcoming the difficulties and fear, the participants will grow. Through overcoming anxious feelings and thoughts outside a person's comfort zone, the individuals will grow (14). At the same time, the debriefing session right after the adventurous experiences can facilitate participants' understanding of the commonly shared meaning of the activity. How the instructor of the ABC framed the activity could enhance individual meaning-making (15).

Voluntary services

Meier and Stutzer (16) stated that voluntary experiences provide the participants with both intrinsic and extrinsic rewards. Intrinsically, the participants feel satisfied by working out the voluntary activities and attain a sense of competence. Extrinsically, the participants' human capital and social network are enhanced and expanded through engaging in the voluntary services. The voluntary experience also provides the participants with social approval, which encourages their prosocial behaviors. Adolescents' sense of civic responsibility is enhanced (17). Other studies also indicate that the prosocial activities like the voluntary services have more positive enhancement on adolescent development than other activities (18). It is evident that the voluntary activities will benefit the adolescents with regard to their sense of responsibility towards the community, positive attitude and behavior (19).

Emotional management group

According to Cherniss et al. (20), emotional intelligence has been linked with a wide range of outcomes in life. Some studies identified the correlation between emotional intelligence and leadership effectiveness. Other studies found the relationship between emotional intelligence and performance in other settings. According to Cavallo and Brienza (21), superior performers in the workplace scored high in all four clusters in emotional intelligence, namely self-awareness, self-management, social awareness and social management. Van Rooy and Viswesvaran (22) investigated the relationship between emotional intelligence and outcomes in different settings by interviewing 69 independent interviewees. The research found a significant linkage ranging from the workplace to educational settings.

OUR STUDY

In 2013, 174 schools were engaged in phase III of the Project, involving 5,042 students. The whole Project was organized in two tiers. Tier 1 was a program for all students while Tier 2 provided services for students with greater psychosocial needs, which were identified by their teachers, parents and/or by self-report questionnaires (23). As reported by the social workers from the participating schools, low social skills, low self-efficacy, self-esteem and difficulties in school adjustment are examples of psychosocial needs encountered by the participants in the Program. Overall, 2,754 participants came from Secondary 1, 888 from Secondary 2 and 1,400 from Secondary 3.

In the sampling process, two social welfare agencies which provide services for six different schools (i.e., one providing services for two schools and another providing for four) were invited. In total, 74 students from these schools joined the focus group interviews. As a longitudinal study, two waves of data collection were conducted. The research team conducted the first wave of data analysis at the end of the first-year program and the second wave one year after the first interview. Table 1 outlines the demographics of the interviewees. Wave 1 interviews were conducted from February to June 2014. There were eight focus groups involving 59 Secondary 1 students from eight different schools. Wave 2 interviews were conducted from May to July 2015, with only three groups including 16 Secondary 2 students from three schools. The other three schools dropped out from Wave 2 data collection due to recruitment problems.

Table 1. Demographic information of interviewees

Wave 1 Group	Total	Male	Female	Wave 2 Total	Male	Female
1	5	0	5	6	0	6
2	7	0	7			
3	8	8	0	5	5	0
4	12	12	0			
5	7	4	3	5	3	2
6*	7	4	3	NIL	NIL	NIL
7*	6	5	1	NIL	NIL	NIL
8*	7	4	3	NIL	NIL	NIL

Note: * Three groups withdrew from wave 2 data collection.

The parental consents were obtained by the agency serving two schools considering that the interviews were held outside the schools. Another agency did not obtain the parental consents as the interviews were scheduled during the normal school hours. Nonetheless, the participants' consents were obtained by the school social workers, who provided the participants with verbal explanations about the purposes, privacy protection measures and procedures of the interviews. The focus group was a semi-structured interview (24). The interviews lasted 60 to 90 minutes. They were conducted by researchers with social work training, who facilitated the participants to express their perceptions and opinions as well as the learning gained from the Program. The entire interview process was audio-taped with the interviewees' consent. The interviewer began with an open invitation, which entailed asking the participants to first recall the program content of the ABA and the social services that they partook in. The participants were then encouraged to reflect upon their experiences.

The participants were facilitated to express their perceptions and opinions in relation to their experience of joining the activities, with the aid of the same interview guide used in the two waves of the longitudinal study. Table 2 shows the different interview questions employed to facilitate the discussions.

Quantitative content analysis was used in this research. According to Margrit Schreier (25), quantitative content analysis denotes the systematic description of coding with the means of coding. It involves the use of a coding frame, generating definitions of categories, and segmenting different materials into the coding units. A frequency count is often employed in the quantitative content analysis. The focus of this type of analysis lies in manifested meaning, contrasting with latent and context-dependent meaning that qualitative content analysis focuses on.

Table 2. Interview questions of the semi-structured group interviews

General Impression of the Program
Do you have any unforgettable experiences about your participation in this program?
Evaluation of the Effectiveness of the Program
Do you think that the program has helped your development?
After participating in the program, do you have any changes? If yes, please specify. (free elicitation)
What have you gained in this program? (free elicitation)
Do you think the program can enhance your abilities in different areas of your life? What are the most useful things that you learned during the process? Can you provide some examples?

Table 3. Comparison of perceived impact between Wave 1 and Wave 2

Perceived Impact	Wave 1 Frequency N = 59	Wave 1 %	Wave 2 Frequency N = 16	Wave 2 %	Chi-square value	df	Contingency coefficient	Level of significance
Improved teamwork	18	31.0	0	0	6.562	1	0.29	0.010**
Built up peer relationships	11	18.9	3	18.9	0	1	0	0.984
Enjoyed the caring spirit	10	17.2	2	12.5	0.207	1	0.05	0.649
Felt satisfied	10	17.2	2	12.5	0.207	1	0.05	0.649
Increased bravery	9	15.5	0	0	2.827	1	0.19	0.093
Enhanced self-confidence	7	12.0	0	0	2.827	1	0.19	0.093
Enhanced communication	5	8.6	4	25	3.149	1	0.2	0.076
Enhanced self-discipline	5	8.6	0	0	1.479	1	0.14	0.224
Learned life skills	5	8.6	0	0	1.479	1	0.14	0.224
Took interpersonal initiative	5	8.6	0	0	1.479	1	0.14	0.224
Improved emotional management	4	6.9	1	3.0	0.008	1	0.01	0.927
Enhanced perception of others	3	5.2	6	18.2	12.268	1	0.38	0.001***
Improved leadership	3	5.2	0	0	1.479	1	0.14	0.224
Became more focused	2	3.4	0	0	0.567	1	0.09	0.451
Became more patient	2	3.4	0	0	0.567	1	0.09	0.451
Improved persistence	2	3.4	0	0	0.567	1	0.09	0.451
Became more careful	1	1.7	0	0	0.28	1	0.06	0.597
Built up a positive self-identity	1	1.7	0	0	0.28	1	0.06	0.597
Enhanced creativity	1	1.7	0	0	0.28	1	0.06	0.597
Enhanced problem-solving skills	1	1.7	2	12.5	3.744	1	0.22	0.053
Enhanced self-understanding	1	1.7	0	0	0.28	1	0.06	0.597
Experienced cooperation	1	1.7	0	0	0.28	1	0.06	0.597
Felt relaxed	1	1.7	0	0	1.167	1	0.13	0.28
Followed instructions	1	1.7	0	0	0.28	1	0.06	0.597
Improved self-determination	1	1.7	9	27.2	31.901	1	0.55	0.001***
Enhanced resilience	0	0	3	18.8	11.335	1	0.36	0.001**
Learned conflict management	0	0	1	6.2	3.675	1	0.22	0.055
Total	110		33					

Note: **$p < 0.05$. ***$p < 0.001$.

Cohen's kappa (26) or k is a measure to calculate how much better than chance the agreement between two coders is. Cohen's kappa is a popular measure of reliability (27). The maximum k value is 1 (100%), which indicates a perfect agreement between the two coders, while the minimum k value is 0, indicating that the agreement is completely different. Viera and Garret (28) classified the rating as Almost Perfect (0.81-0.99); Substantial (0.61-0.80); Moderate (0.41-0.60); Fair (0.21-0.40); and Poor (≤ 0.20).

Chi-square is employed to test whether the distribution of two sets of data is a chance event or not. The greater the significance of this chi-square value is, the less likely that the distribution is due to chance (27). According to Wainer (29), rejecting the null hypothesis and attaining significance at $p < .05$ are satisfactory in the field of social science. In order to answer the research question of this study, the data analysis process included the following steps: (i) coding dialogs in the interviews into different perceived impacts, (ii) counting the frequency of the perceived impacts appearing in each wave, and (iii) comparing the frequency between the two waves using the Pearson's Chi-square analysis. The processed data is presented in Table 3. All of the codings were tagged by one or more activities' names, signaling from which activities the participants attained the coded perceived impacts from the program. This helped to explain the success or failure in the retention of the perceived impact in the later stage.

FINDINGS

After the independent coding was performed by two trained examiners, the agreement between the two coders was tested by Cohen's Kappa test. Three tests were completed as there was a maximum of three perceived impacts coded for the same dialog by the two coders. The results of the three tests are 0.672, 0.679 and 0.854, suggesting either a 'substantial' or an 'almost perfect' level of agreement in the present analysis.

We are able to observe from Table 3 that there are themes mentioned by the respondents in Wave 1 but not in Wave 2. These are improved teamwork (Wave 1: 31%; Wave 2: 0%), increased bravery (Wave 1: 15.5%; Wave 2: 0%), enhanced self-confidence (Wave 1: 12.1%; Wave 2: 0%), enhanced self-discipline and learned life skills (Wave 1: 86.2%; Wave 2: 0%), and taking interpersonal initiative (Wave 1: 86.2%; Wave 2: 0%). On the other hand, there are themes that emerged in both waves but were mentioned more by the respondents in Wave 1 than in Wave 2. These themes are enhanced communication (Wave 1: 8.6%; Wave 2: 2.5%), enjoyed the caring spirit (Wave 1: 17.2%; Wave 2: 12.5%), and felt satisfied (Wave 1: 17.2%; Wave 2: 12.5%). Among these themes, the theme on improved teamwork indicated a statistically significant difference between Waves 1 and 2 ($p < 0.01$). Some of the themes emerged in Wave 1 but were not mentioned by the respondents in Wave 2, and such a discrepancy was statistically significant. These themes included enhanced perception of others ($p < 0.001$) and improved teamwork ($p < 0.01$). Finally, the theme on enhanced resilience (Wave 1: 0%; Wave 2: 18.7%; $p < 0.001$) did not emerge in Wave 1 but was mentioned by the respondents in Wave 2.

Resilience

The findings indicated that the four themes identified by the participants were different in terms of the frequency distribution (all $ps < 0.05$) when comparing the data of Waves 1 and 2. They are (i) Resilience, (ii) Improved teamwork, (iii) Enhanced perception of others, and (iv) Improved self-determination. Comparing the responses of the participants in the two waves, the participants reflected that they were able to enhance their resilience ($p = 0.001$) after joining the second year program. No respondents mentioned this aspect in the Wave 1 data collection. The respondents particularly attributed the enhancement of their resilience to the night walk and camping among the adventurous activities.

"I think the night walk was comparatively useful among all activities which demonstrated greater effectiveness. Before the night walk, our tutors instructed us on how to walk towards the end of the journey, but we felt scared because of the difference between what our tutors instructed us and what the actual situation was like. Nonetheless, even though we were frightened, we started to think of solutions to solve the problems. I think it trained our resilience." (BPS_102)

"I think resilience is also an important thing that this Program wants us to learn; it is related to many things in the camp such as the night walk." (15BPS_94)

Enhanced perception of others

The participants also considered that the Program effectively enhanced their interpersonal skills when they participated in the climbing and camping activities. One participant, who was subjected to rejection by her classmates previously, stated that her classmates became more accepting of her after her participation in the adventurous activities. In a nutshell, the activities enhanced her overall social skills.

"Mutual encouragement. Throughout the process, I understood that competition is not the most important thing. The most important element is to help one another. It is important for me to help others before completing my own task." (BPS1_98)

Strengthened teamwork

Another participant indicated that the climbing activities which required cooperation of the team members enhanced her social skills and teamwork. She learned to listen to others more and not to be dominant when interacting with other students.

> "When we climbed the rock, some people were holding the rope on the ground. We had to communicate because if the pulling force had been too strong or too weak, I would have hit the wall. We learned to talk to each other, to say less about things that people don't fancy listening, to add my own comments only after listening to others, and not to dominate." (BPS_58)

Improved self-determination

The last theme with a statistically significant difference between Wave 1 and Wave 2 is improved self-determination ($p < 0.001$). The night-walk activity was to enhance the participants' self-determination.

> "At the beginning, we walked as a team. Then we had to find a partner to walk with for a while. At the end, we had to walk alone. I think that moment required a certain level of self-determination." (QC2_120)

When comparing the responses of Waves 1 and 2, we could identify several themes regarding which participants had more in-depth description of their experience after one year. The first theme is related to the experience in adventurous training. The participants learned to make decisions and be more courageous when encountering difficulties:

> Wave 1:
> "When we joined the climbing activities, we had to cooperate with our team members. So, I think this Program helped us build up teamwork." (BPS1_173)
> "In the night walk, if we walked with someone we knew, we would feel easier. If we didn't, or if we walked alone, it would be dangerous." (YT_97)
>
> Wave 2:
> "I joined orienteering before. So I think that the feeling of walking at night would be similar. For orienteering, the game result depends on how quickly you accomplish the tasks. Therefore the route that you choose is

decisive. It will affect the result a lot. Similarly, I think that the night walk can help me to become a decisive person." (15BPS_110)

> *"In the night walk, we had to make decisions immediately as to whether we should return along the route we came from or go down the hill along another shorter route. ...So, we had to make decisions immediately. Luckily, we went back to the starting point at the end. Admitting that we were wrong before in choosing the routes, we are thankful that we were decisive and made the decision quickly."* (15BPS_108)

We could see a more in-depth response in Wave 2 than Wave 1. Wave 1 responses are more related to teamwork among the participants while Wave 2 are more related to personal development, including resilience, enhanced perception of others, and improved self-determination. These three themes indicated that the adventurous activities help the participants enhance their social skills which in turn help strengthen their resilience. The respondents talked more about the cooperation among one another in Wave 1 while in Wave 2, they were more able to relate it to their personal development.

The impact of joining voluntary service

Another theme that emerged in Wave 2 but received fewer comments in Wave 1 is the volunteer services that the participants participated in. There is a statistically significant difference ($p < 0.001$) between the frequency of perceived impact counted in Wave 2 than in Wave 1 concerning the voluntary services. The participants learned more about cooperation with others in the volunteer program. One participant talked about an activity involving a social worker which enhanced their teamwork. After the activity, the student learned the importance of being a team member in the volunteer services.

Wave 1:

"I have more patience with the old people and won't find them troublesome. I found them troublesome before this activity because they always put pressure on us. But I don't feel so after doing the voluntary service." (BPS1_78)

"We need to have more empathy and patience towards the old people. Because their hearing has deteriorated, you'd better repeat yourself and do not complain that they are troublesome." (BPS1_80)

Wave 2:
"I could not function well when my eyes were covered. So I realized that when a small part of your body is not functioning well, your life is much affected." (15LKT_45)

Data showing retention of perceived impacts

Another observation from the data indicated that the participants recalled some perceived impact in both waves (Table 3). These are "Building up peer relationships," "Enhanced communication," "Enhanced problem-solving skills," "Enjoying the caring spirit," "Felt satisfied," "Improved conflict management" and "Improved emotional management." There were no statistically significant differences in frequency between Wave 1 and Wave 2. This indicated that the respondents either had strong impressions in regard to these gains after one year or the Program reinforced these impacts in the second year. The responses from the participants indicated that these impacts sustained after one year or reinforced in the second year. This demonstrated the effect in the respondents even after one year.

Data rejecting retention of perceived impacts

A total of 17 themes identified in Wave 1 were not found in Wave 2 (Table 3). These included, for example "Increased bravery," "Enhanced self-discipline," "Learned life skills," "Took interpersonal initiative," "Improved leadership," "Became more focused," "Became more patient," "Improved persistence," "Became more careful," "Built up a positive self-identity", "Enhanced creativity," "Enhanced self-confidence," "Enhanced self-understanding," "Experienced cooperation," and "Feeling relaxed." We can see from the Wave 1 data that the respondents just completed the Program and they had a very fresh memory of the impact of the Program. Therefore, they were more able to talk in detail about the impact of the Program. The building up of peer relationships, communication and conflict management could be seen as part of the elements of the adventurous training and elements of resilience. The respondents were only able to relate to the incident that just occurred but not any incidents about personal growth and development.

DISCUSSION

The results of the present study indicate a strong retention of several constructs one year after completion of the Program. These constructs are mainly related to the team-building and problem-solving activities of the adventurous programs. The participants were able to retain this after one year. This demonstrated the effectiveness of the intervention. The previous longitudinal studies on adolescents' development indicated a strong consistency of those adolescents who have negative or positive schema over time. That is, the adolescents did not demonstrate any statistically significant differences in either positive or negative schema over time. In addition, the negative schema predicts the depressive symptoms among adolescents in second time point of the same longitudinal study (30). The present study indicates similar results that the participants of the Program with a more positive perception of the Program were able to maintain such thoughts over time. Moreover, a previous longitudinal study also indicated that "good interpersonal relationships" are related to the future protective factors of depression in their adulthood (31). The present study in general is consistent with the previous studies and indicates the effectiveness of the

Program that brings about positive interpersonal relationships in relation to feeling satisfied, with more positive problem-solving skills one year after joining the Program.

The data indicates that the adventurous activities facilitate the participants' retention of learning in building up peer relationships, enjoying a caring spirit, enhanced communication, enhanced problem-solving skills as well as improved self-determination. This echoed and reinforced other research findings that the participants obtained psychological benefits from the adventurous activities (13). The participants in the present study were able to benefit from the adventurous activities through various experiential programs and the debriefing by the social workers afterwards. The data of this part further suggested that the volunteer services facilitate the participants' retention of learning in regard to the enhanced perception of others. This reinforces other research findings regarding the participants in the volunteer services (16).

The data suggests that there was a statistically significant difference between the frequency of "improved teamwork" in Wave 1 and Wave 2. The failure of retention is likely to be due to the difference in nature between improved teamwork and the other three perceived impacts (enhanced adversity quotient, improved self-determination and enhanced perception of others). Teamwork is a kind of learning dependent on the emotional bonding among the groups (32), while the other three are not. Therefore, upon completion of the group activities, the participants reported their perceived impact of teamwork in the Wave 1 interviews. However, between the Wave 1 and Wave 2 interviews, without any programs strengthening the emotional bonding among the group members, no participants mentioned their learning of teamwork. This reveals a failure of retention of improved teamwork as a perceived impact. Nevertheless, we were able to capture a more in-depth reflection on the effects of the Program to allow a more sophisticated understanding of enhanced resilience. This observation was also consistent with the literature on prosocial responding and moral reasoning. A previous study indicated the development of adolescents' prosocial and moral reasoning in their developmental processes. There will be an increase in moral reasoning until their early 20s (33). Together with the cognitive development of the adolescents, their way of perceiving the impact of the Program became more sophisticated and more generalized into their daily life.

Limitations of the study

The present study has a few limitations. First, the number of interviewees was not equal in the two waves of interviews although a suitable data analysis method was employed to minimize the effect of this inequality. Second, details in relation to the program activities run by different schools between the Wave 1 and Wave 2 interviews were unknown, which might affect the retention of the perceived impact. Nonetheless, the current study has offered a reasonable hypothesis and explanation for the general effect of the activities between the two waves. The adventurous programs together with the volunteer activities were able to enhance their positive youth development over a year. In particular, the adventurous programs indicated a higher impact on the participants' perception of the effect of the Program in their life. This study also demonstrated an in-depth consolidation of the experience after one year in some participants.

Acknowledgments

The Project P.A.T.H.S. and the preparation for this paper were financially supported by The Hong Kong Jockey Club Charities Trust. This paper is based on an article published in the International Journal on Disability and Human Development 2018;17(3) issue. We thank the participants for joining this study.

REFERENCES

[1] Catalano RF, Berglund ML, Ryan JAM, Lonczak HS, Hawkins JD. Positive youth development in the United States: Research findings on evaluations of positive youth development programs. Prev Treat 2002;5(1):Article 15. DOI: 10.1037/1522-3736.5.1.515a.

[2] Shek DTL, Sun RCF. Implementation of the tier 1 program of the project PATHS: Interim evaluation findings. ScientificWorldJournal 2006;6:2274-84.

[3] Shek DTL, Ma HK. Subjective outcome evaluation of the Project P.A.T.H.S.: Findings based on the perspective of the program participants. Scientific WorldJournal 2007;7:47-55.

[4] Shek DTL, Siu AMH, Lee TY. Subjective outcome evaluation of the project P.A.T.H.S.: Findings based on the perspective of the program implementers. ScientificWorldJournal 2007;7:195-203.

[5] Shek DTL, Ma HK, Sun RCF. Interim evaluation of the tier 1 program (secondary 1 curriculum) of the Project P.A.T.H.S.: First year of the full implementation phase. ScientificWorldJournal 2008;8:47-60.

[6] Shek DTL, Ma HK, Sun RCF, Lung DWM. Process evaluation of the tier 1 program (secondary 1 curriculum) of Project P.A.T.H.S.: Findings based on the full implementation phase. ScientificWorldJournal 2008;8:35-46.

[7] Shek DTL, Yu L. Prevention of adolescent problem behavior: Longitudinal impact of the Project P.A.T.H.S. in Hong Kong. ScientificWorldJournal 2011;11:546-67.

[8] Shek DTL, Ma CMS. Impact of the Project P.A.T.H.S. in the junior secondary school years: Objective outcome evaluation based on eight waves of longitudinal data. ScientificWorldJournal 2012;2012:Article ID 170345. DOI: 10.1100/2012/170345.

[9] Campbell DT, Stanley JC. Experimental and quasi-experimental designs for research. Ravenio Books, 2015.

[10] Shek DTL, Yu L. Longitudinal impact of the Project P.A.T.H.S. on adolescent risk behavior: What happened after five years? ScientificWorldJournal 2012;2012:Article ID 316029. DOI: 10.1100/2012/316029.

[11] Shek DTL, Ng CSM. Early identification of adolescents with greater psychosocial needs: An evaluation of the Project P.A.T.H.S. in Hong Kong. Int J Disabil Hum Dev 2010;9(4):291-9.

[12] Fletcher TB, Hinkle S. Adventure based counselling: An innovation in counselling. J Couns Dev 2002;80:277-85.

[13] Kyriakopoulos A. Adventure based counselling, individual counselling and object relations: A critical evaluation of a qualitative study. Eur J Psychother Couns 2010;12(4):311-22.

[14] Luckner JL, Nadler RS. Processing the experience: Strategies to enhance and generalize learning, 2nd ed. Dubuque, IA: Kendall Hunt, 1997.

[15] Long AE. Learning the ropes: Exploring the meaning and value of experiential education for girls at risk. J Experiential Educ 2001;24(2):100-8.
[16] Meier S, Stutzer A. Is volunteering rewarding in itself? Economica 2008;75(297): 39-59.
[17] Schmidt JA, Shumow L, Kackar H. Adolescents' participation in service activities and its impact on academic, behavioral, and civic outcomes. J Youth Adolesc 2007;36(2):127-40.
[18] Hansen DM, Larson RW, Dworkin JB. What adolescents learn in organized youth activities: A survey of self-reported developmental experiences. J Res Adolsec 2003;13(1):25-55.
[19] Zeldin S. Preventing youth violence through the promotion of community engagement and membership. J Commun Psychol 2004;32(5):623-41.
[20] Cherniss C, Extein M, Goleman D, Weissberg RP. Emotional intelligence: What does the research really indicate? Educ Psychol 2006;41(4):239-45. DOI: 10.1207/s15326985ep4104_4.
[21] Cavallo K, Brienza D. Emotional competence and leadership excellence at Johnson & Johnson: The emotional intelligence and leadership study. New Brunswick, NJ: Consortium for Research on Emotional Intelligence in Organizations, Rutgers, 2004.
[22] Van Rooy DL, Viswesvaran C. Emotional intelligence: A meta-analytic investigation of predictive validity and nomological net. J Vocat Behav 2004;65: 71-95.
[23] Shek DTL, Ma HK. Design of a positive youth development program in Hong Kong. Int J Adolesc Med Health 2006;18(3):315-28.
[24] Smith JA, Osborn M. Pain as an assault on the self: An interpretative phenomenological analysis of the psychological impact of chronic benign low back pain. Psychol Health. 2007;22(5):517-34.
[25] Schreier M. Qualitative content analysis. In: Flick, U, ed. The Sage handbook of qualitative data analysis. Thousand Oaks, CA: Sage, 2013:170-83.
[26] Cohen J. A coefficient of agreement for nominal scales. Educ Psychol Meas 1960;20:37-46.
[27] Bernard HR, Bernard HR. Social research methods: Qualitative and quantitative approaches, 2nd ed. Thousand Oaks, CA: Sage, 2013.
[28] Viera AJ, Garrett JM. Understanding interobserver agreement: The kappa statistic. Fam Med 2005;37(5):360-3.
[29] Wainer H. One cheer for null hypothesis significance testing. Psychol Methods 1999;4(2):212-3.
[30] Friedmann JS, Lumley MN, Lerman B. Cognitive schemas as longitudinal predictors of self-reported adolescent depressive symptoms and resilience. Cogn Behav Ther 2016;45(1):32-48.
[31] Carbonell DM, Reinherz HZ, Giaconia RM, Stashwick CK, Paradis AD, Beardslee WR. Adolescent protective factors promoting resilience in young adults at risk for depression. Child Adolesc Soc Work J 2002;19(5):393-412.

[32] Graen GB. Excellence in socio-technical teamwork requires both cognitive and emotional bonding. Am Psychol 2009;64(1):52-3.

[33] Eisenberg N, Cumberland A, Guthrie IK, Murphy BC, Shepard SA. Age changes in prosocial responding and moral reasoning in adolescence and early adulthood. J Res Adolesc 2005;15(3):235-60.

SECTION TWO: ACKNOWLEDGMENTS

In: Psychosocial Needs
Editors: Daniel TL Shek et al.

ISBN: 978-1-53611-951-0
© 2017 Nova Science Publishers, Inc.

Chapter 12

ABOUT THE EDITORS

Daniel TL Shek PhD, FHKPS, BBS, SBS, JP is Associate Vice President (Undergraduate Programme) and Chair Professor of Applied Social Sciences at The Hong Kong Polytechnic University. He is also Advisory Professor of East China Normal University and Adjunct Professor of University of Kentucky College of Medicine. He is Chief Editor of *Journal of Youth Studies* and *Applied Research in Quality of Life*, Associate Editor of *Frontier in Child Health and Human Development* and past Consulting Editor of *Journal of Clinical Psychology*. He is a Series Editor of *Quality of Life in Asia* published by Springer. He is an Editorial Advisor of *The British Journal of Social Work* and an Editorial Board member of eight international journals, including *Social Indicators Research, Journal of Adolescent Health* and *Journal of Child and Family Studies*. Professor Shek has to date published 144 books, 394 book chapters and more than 650 articles in international refereed journals. Email: daniel.shek@polyu.edu.hk

Janet TY Leung, MA, PhD, is an Assistant Professor of the Department of Applied Social Sciences at The Hong Kong Polytechnic University. She is a registered social worker and has been working in the social welfare field for over 20 years. She was a service supervisor in a social service organization and was responsible to supervise a wide range of services, such as children and youth services, school counseling services, training projects for dyslexic children, family support programs, service for the homeless people and community development projects. Her areas of interests include poverty, adolescent development, family processes and parent education. Email: janet.leung@polyu.edu.hk

Tak Yan Lee, MSW, PhD, is an Associate Professor of the Department of Applied Social Sciences at The City University of Hong Kong. His teaching and research interests are in group work, positive youth development, and practice teaching and learning. His research covers adolescent prostitution, positive youth development, parent–child communication, parental control, and resilience of children and the elderly. He had provided consultancy to statutory bodies and social service agencies on civic awareness, youth development indices, moral values and behavior, sociocultural beliefs, gambling behavior, and compensated dating. He had also conducted research on fieldwork learning strategy and field instruction. Email: ty.lee@cityu.edu.hk

Joav Merrick, MD, MMedSci, DMSc, born and educated in Denmark is professor of pediatrics, child health and human development, Division of Pediatrics, Hadassah Hebrew University Medical Center, Mt Scopus Campus, Jerusalem, Israel and Kentucky Children's Hospital, University of Kentucky, Lexington, Kentucky, United States and professor of public health at the Center for Healthy Development, School of Public Health, Georgia State University, Atlanta, United States, the medical director of the Health Services, Division for Intellectual and Developmental Disabilities, Ministry of Social Affairs and Social Services, Jerusalem, the founder and director of the National Institute of Child Health and Human Development in Israel. He has numerous publications in the field of pediatrics, child health and human development, rehabilitation, intellectual disability, disability, health, welfare, abuse, advocacy, quality of life and prevention. He received the Peter Sabroe

Child Award for outstanding work on behalf of Danish Children in 1985 and the International LEGO-Prize ("The Children's Nobel Prize") for an extraordinary contribution towards improvement in child welfare and well-being in 1987. Email: jmerrick@zahav.net.il

In: Psychosocial Needs
Editors: Daniel TL Shek et al.
ISBN: 978-1-53611-951-0
© 2017 Nova Science Publishers, Inc.

Chapter 13

ABOUT THE DEPARTMENT OF APPLIED SOCIAL SCIENCES, THE HONG KONG POLYTECHNIC UNIVERSITY, HUNGHOM, HONG KONG

The Department of Applied Social Sciences (APSS) of the Hong Kong Polytechnic University began as the Institute of Social Work Training in 1973 before it became the School of Social Work in the Hong Kong Polytechnic in 1977. In 2000, six years after the Polytechnic became a university, the department was renamed as the Department of Applied Social Sciences. It is now one of the largest social science departments in the Asia-Pacific region with a strong tradition of researching on and working with socially vulnerable groups through education, research and service in diverse areas incorporating social work, social policy and administration, psychology, sociology and philosophy.

Education

In education, we strive to nurture human service professionals who are knowledgeable, resourceful, caring, worldly but reflexive, and possess a strong commitment to social justice and responsibility. We also see them as practitioners and researchers who are able to integrate theory and practice, and develop appropriate indigenous knowledge that can meet the challenges of rapid social change in Chinese societies.

Research

In research, to respond to the constantly changing global socio-economic order and addressing the subsequently emerged local problems, the strategic foci of our research and social investigation have also been expanded to include migration and mobilities, family and life-span development, social economy, online communities/social media, disaster and risks reduction, applied philosophy and social work practices.

Community service

In community service, we continue to collaborate with community partners to allow our students to understand better the different lifeworlds of our society, design programmes and supportive services that are innovative, relevant and socially responsible.

Students

As for students in our department, we see it necessary for them to develop a global outlook while firmly grounded in Hong Kong. To this end, in recent years more than 200 full-time and part-time students as well as alumni have participated in the various study tours and exchange programmes we held in the Chinese Mainland and overseas, including the University of Nottingham, United Kingdom; University of Queensland, Australia; University of California at Berkeley, United States; Washington

University in St. Louis, United States; York University, Canada; Peking University and Yunnan University in China.

Faculty and teaching

In the 2016/17 academic year, the Department has about 250 members, including academic staff, part-time fieldwork instructors, research and project staff and administrative and supporting technical staff. The APSS offers nearly 18 undergraduate and coursework and research postgraduate programmes with an annual enrolment number of about 1,200 students and over the years more than 17,000 students have graduated.

In: Psychosocial Needs
Editors: Daniel TL Shek et al.

ISBN: 978-1-53611-951-0
© 2017 Nova Science Publishers, Inc.

Chapter 14

ABOUT THE NATIONAL INSTITUTE OF CHILD HEALTH AND HUMAN DEVELOPMENT IN ISRAEL

The National Institute of Child Health and Human Development (NICHD) in Israel was established in 1998 as a virtual institute under the auspices of the Medical Director, Ministry of Social Affairs and Social Services in order to function as the research arm for the Office of the Medical Director. In 1998 the National Council for Child Health and Pediatrics, Ministry of Health and in 1999 the Director General and Deputy Director General of the Ministry of Health endorsed the establishment of the NICHD.

Mission

The mission of a National Institute for Child Health and Human Development in Israel is to provide an academic focal point for the scholarly interdisciplinary study of child life, health, public health, welfare, disability, rehabilitation, intellectual disability and related aspects of human development. This mission includes research, teaching, clinical work, information and public service activities in the field of child health and human development.

Service and academic activities

Over the years many activities became focused in the south of Israel due to collaboration with various professionals at the Faculty of Health Sciences (FOHS) at the Ben Gurion University of the Negev (BGU). Since 2000 an affiliation with the Zusman Child Development Center at the Pediatric Division of Soroka University Medical Center has resulted in collaboration around the establishment of the Down Syndrome Clinic at that center. In 2002 a full course on "Disability" was established at the Recanati School for Allied Professions in the Community, FOHS, BGU and in 2005 collaboration was started with the Primary Care Unit of the faculty and disability became part of the master of public health course on "Children and society". In the academic year 2005-2006 a one semester course on "Aging with disability" was started as part of the master of science program in gerontology in our collaboration with the Center for Multidisciplinary Research in Aging. In 2010 collaborations with the Division of Pediatrics, Hadassah Hebrew University Medical Center, Jerusalem, Israel around the National Down Syndrome Center and teaching students and residents about intellectual and developmental disabilities as part of their training at this campus.

Research activities

The affiliated staff have over the years published work from projects and research activities in this national and international collaboration. In the year 2000 the International Journal of Adolescent Medicine and Health and in 2005 the International Journal on Disability and Human Development of

De Gruyter Publishing House (Berlin and New York) were affiliated with the National Institute of Child Health and Human Development. From 2008 also the International Journal of Child Health and Human Development (Nova Science, New York), the International Journal of Child and Adolescent Health (Nova Science) and the Journal of Pain Management (Nova Science) affiliated and from 2009 the International Public Health Journal (Nova Science) and Journal of Alternative Medicine Research (Nova Science). All peer-reviewed international journals.

National collaborations

Nationally the NICHD works in collaboration with the Faculty of Health Sciences, Ben Gurion University of the Negev; Department of Physical Therapy, Sackler School of Medicine, Tel Aviv University; Autism Center, Assaf HaRofeh Medical Center; National Rett and PKU Centers at Chaim Sheba Medical Center, Tel HaShomer; Department of Physiotherapy, Haifa University; Department of Education, BarIlan University, Ramat Gan, Faculty of Social Sciences and Health Sciences; College of Judea and Samaria in Ariel and in 2011 affiliation with Center for Pediatric Chronic Diseases and National Center for Down Syndrome, Department of Pediatrics, Hadassah Hebrew University Medical Center, Mount Scopus Campus, Jerusalem.

International collaborations

Internationally with the Department of Disability and Human Development, College of Applied Health Sciences, University of Illinois at Chicago; Strong Center for Developmental Disabilities, Golisano Children's Hospital at Strong, University of Rochester School of Medicine and Dentistry, New York; Centre on Intellectual Disabilities, University of Albany, New York; Centre for Chronic Disease Prevention and Control,

Health Canada, Ottawa; Chandler Medical Center and Children's Hospital, Kentucky Children's Hospital, Section of Adolescent Medicine, University of Kentucky, Lexington; Chronic Disease Prevention and Control Research Center, Baylor College of Medicine, Houston, Texas; Division of Neuroscience, Department of Psychiatry, Columbia University, New York; Institute for the Study of Disadvantage and Disability, Atlanta; Center for Autism and Related Disorders, Department Psychiatry, Children's Hospital Boston, Boston; Department of Pediatric and Adolescent Medicine, Western Michigan University Homer Stryker MD School of Medicine, Kalamazoo, Michigan, United States; Department of Paediatrics, Child Health and Adolescent Medicine, Children's Hospital at Westmead, Westmead, Australia; International Centre for the Study of Occupational and Mental Health, Düsseldorf, Germany; Centre for Advanced Studies in Nursing, Department of General Practice and Primary Care, University of Aberdeen, Aberdeen, United Kingdom; Quality of Life Research Center, Copenhagen, Denmark; Nordic School of Public Health, Gottenburg, Sweden, Scandinavian Institute of Quality of Working Life, Oslo, Norway; The Department of Applied Social Sciences (APSS) of The Hong Kong Polytechnic University Hong Kong.

Targets

Our focus is on research, international collaborations, clinical work, teaching and policy in health, disability and human development and to establish the NICHD as a permanent institute in Israel in order to conduct model research and together with the four university schools of public health/medicine in Israel establish a national master and doctoral program in disability and human development at the institute to secure the next generation of professionals working in this often non-prestigious/low-status field of work.

Contact

Joav Merrick, MD, MMedSci, DMSc
Professor of Pediatrics
Medical Director, Health Services, Division for Intellectual and Developmental Disabilities, Ministry of Social Affairs and Social Services, POB 1260, IL-91012 Jerusalem, Israel.
E-mail: jmerrick@zahav.net.il

In: Psychosocial Needs
Editors: Daniel TL Shek et al.

ISBN: 978-1-53611-951-0
© 2017 Nova Science Publishers, Inc.

Chapter 15

ABOUT THE BOOK SERIES "HEALTH AND HUMAN DEVELOPMENT"

Health and human development is a book series with publications from a multidisciplinary group of researchers, practitioners and clinicians for an international professional forum interested in the broad spectrum of health and human development. Books already published:

- Merrick J, Omar HA, eds. Adolescent behavior research. International perspectives. New York: Nova Science, 2007.
- Kratky KW. Complementary medicine systems: Comparison and integration. New York: Nova Science, 2008.
- Schofield P, Merrick J, eds. Pain in children and youth. New York: Nova Science, 2009.
- Greydanus DE, Patel DR, Pratt HD, Calles Jr JL, eds. Behavioral pediatrics, 3 ed. New York: Nova Science, 2009.
- Ventegodt S, Merrick J, eds. Meaningful work: Research in quality of working life. New York: Nova Science, 2009.
- Omar HA, Greydanus DE, Patel DR, Merrick J, eds. Obesity and adolescence. A public health concern. New York: Nova Science, 2009.
- Lieberman A, Merrick J, eds. Poverty and children. A public health concern. New York: Nova Science, 2009.

- Goodbread J. Living on the edge. The mythical, spiritual and philosophical roots of social marginality. New York: Nova Science, 2009.
- Bennett DL, Towns S, Elliot E, Merrick J, eds. Challenges in adolescent health: An Australian perspective. New York: Nova Science, 2009.
- Schofield P, Merrick J, eds. Children and pain. New York: Nova Science, 2009.
- Sher L, Kandel I, Merrick J, eds. Alcohol-related cognitive disorders: Research and clinical perspectives. New York: Nova Science, 2009.
- Anyanwu EC. Advances in environmental health effects of toxigenic mold and mycotoxins. New York: Nova Science, 2009.
- Bell E, Merrick J, eds. Rural child health. International aspects. New York: Nova Science, 2009.
- Dubowitz H, Merrick J, eds. International aspects of child abuse and neglect. New York: Nova Science, 2010.
- Shahtahmasebi S, Berridge D. Conceptualizing behavior: A practical guide to data analysis. New York: Nova Science, 2010.
- Wernik U. Chance action and therapy. The playful way of changing. New York: Nova Science, 2010.
- Omar HA, Greydanus DE, Patel DR, Merrick J, eds. Adolescence and chronic illness. A public health concern. New York: Nova Science, 2010.
- Patel DR, Greydanus DE, Omar HA, Merrick J, eds. Adolescence and sports. New York: Nova Science, 2010.
- Shek DTL, Ma HK, Merrick J, eds. Positive youth development: Evaluation and future directions in a Chinese context. New York: Nova Science, 2010.
- Shek DTL, Ma HK, Merrick J, eds. Positive youth development: Implementation of a youth program in a Chinese context. New York: Nova Science, 2010.
- Omar HA, Greydanus DE, Tsitsika AK, Patel DR, Merrick J, eds. Pediatric and adolescent sexuality and gynecology: Principles for the primary care clinician. New York: Nova Science, 2010.
- Chow E, Merrick J, eds. Advanced cancer. Pain and quality of life. New York: Nova Science, 2010.
- Latzer Y, Merrick, J, Stein D, eds. Understanding eating disorders. Integrating culture, psychology and biology. New York: Nova Science, 2010.

About the book series "Health and human development" 247

- Sahgal A, Chow E, Merrick J, eds. Bone and brain metastases: Advances in research and treatment. New York: Nova Science, 2010.
- Postolache TT, Merrick J, eds. Environment, mood disorders and suicide. New York: Nova Science, 2010.
- Maharajh HD, Merrick J, eds. Social and cultural psychiatry experience from the Caribbean Region. New York: Nova Science, 2010.
- Mirsky J. Narratives and meanings of migration. New York: Nova Science, 2010.
- Harvey PW. Self-management and the health care consumer. New York: Nova Science, 2011.
- Ventegodt S, Merrick J. Sexology from a holistic point of view. New York: Nova Science, 2011.
- Ventegodt S, Merrick J. Principles of holistic psychiatry: A textbook on holistic medicine for mental disorders. New York: Nova Science, 2011.
- Greydanus DE, Calles Jr JL, Patel DR, Nazeer A, Merrick J, eds. Clinical aspects of psychopharmacology in childhood and adolescence. New York: Nova Science, 2011.
- Bell E, Seidel BM, Merrick J, eds. Climate change and rural child health. New York: Nova Science, 2011.
- Bell E, Zimitat C, Merrick J, eds. Rural medical education: Practical strategies. New York: Nova Science, 2011.
- Latzer Y, Tzischinsky. The dance of sleeping and eating among adolescents: Normal and pathological perspectives. New York: Nova Science, 2011.
- Deshmukh VD. The astonishing brain and holistic consciousness: Neuroscience and Vedanta perspectives. New York: Nova Science, 2011.
- Bell E, Westert GP, Merrick J, eds. Translational research for primary healthcare. New York: Nova Science, 2011.
- Shek DTL, Sun RCF, Merrick J, eds. Drug abuse in Hong Kong: Development and evaluation of a prevention program. New York: Nova Science, 2011.
- Ventegodt S, Hermansen TD, Merrick J. Human Development: Biology from a holistic point of view. New York: Nova Science, 2011.
- Ventegodt S, Merrick J. Our search for meaning in life. New York: Nova Science, 2011.

- Caron RM, Merrick J, eds. Building community capacity: Minority and immigrant populations. New York: Nova Science, 2012.
- Klein H, Merrick J, eds. Human immunodeficiency virus (HIV) research: Social science aspects. New York: Nova Science, 2012.
- Lutzker JR, Merrick J, eds. Applied public health: Examining multifaceted Social or ecological problems and child maltreatment. New York: Nova Science, 2012.
- Chemtob D, Merrick J, eds. AIDS and tuberculosis: Public health aspects. New York: Nova Science, 2012.
- Ventegodt S, Merrick J. Textbook on evidence-based holistic mind-body medicine: Basic principles of healing in traditional Hippocratic medicine. New York: Nova Science, 2012.
- Ventegodt S, Merrick J. Textbook on evidence-based holistic mind-body medicine: Holistic practice of traditional Hippocratic medicine. New York: Nova Science, 2012.
- Ventegodt S, Merrick J. Textbook on evidence-based holistic mind-body medicine: Healing the mind in traditional Hippocratic medicine. New York: Nova Science, 2012.
- Ventegodt S, Merrick J. Textbook on evidence-based holistic mind-body medicine: Sexology and traditional Hippocratic medicine. New York: Nova Science, 2012.
- Ventegodt S, Merrick J. Textbook on evidence-based holistic mind-body medicine: Research, philosophy, economy and politics of traditional Hippocratic medicine. New York: Nova Science, 2012.
- Caron RM, Merrick J, eds. Building community capacity: Skills and principles. New York: Nova Science, 2012.
- Lemal M, Merrick J, eds. Health risk communication. New York: Nova Science, 2012.
- Ventegodt S, Merrick J. Textbook on evidence-based holistic mind-body medicine: Basic philosophy and ethics of traditional Hippocratic medicine. New York: Nova Science, 2013.
- Caron RM, Merrick J, eds. Building community capacity: Case examples from around the world. New York: Nova Science, 2013.
- Steele RE. Managed care in a public setting. New York: Nova Science, 2013.
- Srabstein JC, Merrick J, eds. Bullying: A public health concern. New York: Nova Science, 2013.
- Pulenzas N, Lechner B, Thavarajah N, Chow E, Merrick J, eds. Advanced cancer: Managing symptoms and quality of life. New York: Nova Science, 2013.

- Stein D, Latzer Y, eds. Treatment and recovery of eating disorders. New York: Nova Science, 2013.
- Sun J, Buys N, Merrick J. Health promotion: Community singing as a vehicle to promote health. New York: Nova Science, 2013.
- Pulenzas N, Lechner B, Thavarajah N, Chow E, Merrick J, eds. Advanced cancer: Managing symptoms and quality of life. New York: Nova Science, 2013.
- Sun J, Buys N, Merrick J. Health promotion: Strengthening positive health and preventing disease. New York: Nova Science, 2013.
- Merrick J, Israeli S, eds. Food, nutrition and eating behavior. New York: Nova Science, 2013.
- Shahtahmasebi S, Merrick J. Suicide from a public health perspective.
  New York: Nova Science, 2014.
- Merrick J, Tenenbaum A, eds. Public health concern: Smoking, alcohol and substance use. New York: Nova Science, 2014.
- Merrick J, Aspler S, Morad M, eds. Mental health from an international perspective. New York: Nova Science, 2014.
- Merrick J, ed. India: Health and human development aspects. New York: Nova Science, 2014.
- Caron R, Merrick J, eds. Public health: Improving health via inter-professional collaborations. New York: Nova Science, 2014.
- Merrick J, ed. Pain Mangement Yearbook 2014. New York: Nova Science, 2015.
- Merrick J, ed. Public Health Yearbook 2014. New York: Nova Science, 2015.
- Sher L, Merrick J, eds. Forensic psychiatry: A public health perspective. New York: Nova Science, 2015.
- Shek DTL, Wu FKY, Merrick J, eds. Leadership and service learning education: Holistic development for Chinese university students. New York: Nova Science, 2015.
- Calles JL, Greydanus DE, Merrick J, eds. Mental and holistic health: Some international perspectives. New York: Nova Science, 2015.
- Lechner B, Chow R, Pulenzas N, Popovic M, Zhang N, Zhang X, Chow E, Merrick J, eds. Cancer: Treatment, decision making and quality of life. New York: Nova Science, 2016.
- Lechner B, Chow R, Pulenzas N, Popovic M, Zhang N, Zhang X, Chow E, Merrick J, eds. Cancer: Pain and symptom management. New York: Nova Science, 2016.

- Lechner B, Chow R, Pulenzas N, Popovic M, Zhang N, Zhang X, Chow E, Merrick J, eds. Cancer: Bone metastases, CNS metastases and pathological fractures. New York: Nova Science, 2016.
- Lechner B, Chow R, Pulenzas N, Popovic M, Zhang N, Zhang X, Chow E, Merrick J, eds. Cancer: Spinal cord, lung, breast, cervical, prostate, head and neck cancer. New York: Nova Science, 2016.
- Lechner B, Chow R, Pulenzas N, Popovic M, Zhang N, Zhang X, Chow E, Merrick J, eds. Cancer: Survival, quality of life and ethical implications. New York: Nova Science, 2016.
- Davidovitch N, Gross Z, Ribakov Y, Slobodianiuk A, eds. Quality, mobility and globalization in the higher education system: A comparative look at the challenges of academic teaching. New York: Nova Science, 2016.
- Henry B, Agarwal A, Chow E, Omar HA, Merrick J, eds. Cannabis: Medical aspects. New York: Nova Science, 2017.
- Henry B, Agarwal A, Chow E, Merrick J, eds. Palliative care: Psychosocial and ethical considerations. New York: Nova Science, 2017.
- Furfari A, Charames GS, McDonald R, Rowbottom L, Azad A, Chan S, Wan BA, Chow R, DeAngelis C, Zaki P, Chow E, Merrick J, eds. Oncology: The promising future of biomarkers. New York: Nova Science, 2017.

Contact

Professor Joav Merrick, MD, MMedSci, DMSc
Medical Director, Health Services
Division for Intellectual and Developmental Disabilities
Ministry of Social Affairs and Social Services
PO Box 1260, IL-91012 Jerusalem, Israel
E-mail: jmerrick@zahav.net.il

SECTION THREE: INDEX

INDEX

A

abstract conceptualization, 113, 196, 202, 204, 206
academic ability grouping, 195, 197, 202, 203, 204
academic motivation, 146
academic performance, 61, 109, 134, 146, 147, 150, 201, 203
academic skills, 204, 207
academic success, 70
academic underachievement, 146, 166
accountability, 212
achievement orientation, 207
achievement test, 197
action taken, 196, 198, 200, 202
active experimentation, 113, 198
actual participation, 200
adjustment, 56, 91, 118, 141, 165
administrative support, 91
adolescent behavior, 147
adolescent development, 2, 10, 26, 32, 63, 65, 71, 81, 94, 102, 114, 168, 212, 232
adolescent guidance, 138
adolescent problem behavior(s), 147, 171, 226

adolescent risk behavior, 2, 3, 226
adolescents, xv, xxii, 1, 2, 3, 4, 5, 6, 9, 10, 11, 12, 13, 16, 17, 21, 22, 23, 29, 30, 32, 41, 44, 47, 48, 51, 52, 65, 69, 70, 72, 73, 74, 75, 76, 82, 92, 94, 95, 97, 98, 99, 102, 109, 113, 115, 120, 121, 122, 123, 124, 138, 139, 140, 142, 143, 145, 146, 147, 149, 162, 163, 164, 166, 167, 168, 170, 186, 187, 191, 192, 196, 200, 207, 209, 211, 213, 223, 224, 226, 227, 247
adulthood, 10, 147, 164, 168, 223, 228
adults, 11, 12, 22, 98, 127
adventure-based, 4, 14, 52, 75, 81, 100, 103, 104, 105, 106, 113, 124, 126, 132, 139, 148, 149, 152, 162, 163, 167, 171, 179, 196, 203, 211
adventure-based activities, 75, 81, 103, 171, 179, 196, 203
adventure-based counseling, 4, 113, 124, 148, 149, 152, 162, 163
adventure-based training, 100, 103, 104, 106, 113, 124, 132, 139
affective relationship, 188
aggression, 10
alcohol, ix, xvi
altruism, 180

anger, 154, 157
antisocial behavior, 146
anxiety, 99, 146, 212
application, 6, 43, 107, 119, 126, 170, 171, 174, 179, 189, 190, 191, 204
arthritis, 192
articulation, 99
Asia, 207, 208, 231, 235
aspiration, 106, 110
assessment, 43, 132, 163, 197, 207
assets, 11, 95, 99, 123, 147, 164
atmosphere, 10, 20, 23, 60, 92, 151
at-risk populations, 193
attachment, 187, 192
attitude(s), 35, 37, 44, 49, 51, 55, 74, 75, 78, 81, 85, 90, 91, 100, 110, 113, 123, 131, 151, 162, 167, 170, 180, 207, 213
awareness, 19, 22, 44, 51, 61, 74, 81, 82, 100, 124, 182, 213, 232

B

behavioral, 22, 52, 61, 71, 72, 78, 89, 91, 123, 146, 147, 152, 161, 162, 166, 170, 176, 180, 182, 184, 186, 196, 198, 204, 207, 210, 212, 227
behavioral changes, 182
behavioral competence, 52, 71, 72, 78, 123, 152, 161, 170, 176, 184, 186, 210
behavioral problems, 162
behavioral sciences, 207
behavioral self-regulation, 204
behaviors, 44, 49, 60, 62, 75, 85, 89, 146, 147, 153, 167, 172
beliefs in the future, 10, 18, 123, 152, 170, 210
beneficial effect, 30
benefits, xxii, 4, 5, 11, 18, 31, 32, 40, 43, 44, 90, 119, 121, 122, 124, 127, 128, 129, 137, 139, 146, 152, 153, 158, 161, 163, 164, 224

bonding, 16, 17, 52, 123, 152, 155, 170, 176, 183, 184, 187, 193, 210, 224, 228
building blocks, 51, 123
bullying, 146, 179

C

cancer, viii, xiii, 246, 248, 249
Cantonese, 17, 197
career counseling, 114, 119, 123
career development, xxii, 98, 99, 100, 101, 102, 112, 113, 114, 115, 119, 121, 122, 123, 124, 125, 127, 128, 137, 138, 139, 142
career guidance, 99, 114, 119
caregivers, 11, 187
caring, 22, 23, 27, 30, 41, 74, 75, 78, 81, 83, 90, 110, 114, 123, 142, 159, 164, 179, 216, 218, 222, 224, 235
case study, 5, 26, 41, 210
catalyst, 112
category a, 150
causal attribution, 66
causal relationship, 189
challenges, 11, 19, 22, 50, 56, 81, 91, 119, 131, 138, 143, 147, 155, 162, 184, 236, 250
changing environment, 99
chaos, 103, 138
child abuse, 246
child maltreatment, 248
childhood, 2, 166, 192, 247
children, 10, 26, 32, 44, 52, 142, 155, 159, 167, 168, 184, 192, 207, 232, 245
China, 1, 9, 14, 29, 47, 69, 97, 119, 121, 145, 150, 169, 195, 209, 231, 237
Chinese, v, xiii, 4, 6, 11, 24, 25, 30, 40, 41, 48, 70, 95, 119, 122, 142, 143, 146, 147, 167, 188, 191, 192, 193, 197, 199, 207, 208, 236, 246, 249

classroom, 21, 33, 40, 44, 59, 89, 101, 164, 166, 196
clear and positive identity, 52, 72, 78, 123, 152, 171, 210
clinical depression, 32, 43
close relationships, 92
coding, 17, 102, 128, 152, 170, 175, 176, 196, 201, 202, 215, 217
cognitive competence, 123, 128, 152, 161, 170, 184, 210
cognitive development, 225
cognitive dysfunction, 31
cognitive function, 30, 42
cognitive impairment, 31
collaboration, 4, 88, 92, 99, 240, 241
commitment, 27, 74, 75, 78, 91, 187, 236
communication, 20, 39, 52, 56, 57, 72, 73, 75, 78, 80, 81, 82, 96, 110, 122, 127, 133, 134, 137, 154, 155, 156, 158, 179, 180, 181, 182, 186, 188, 216, 218, 222, 223, 224, 232, 248
communication skills, 20, 39, 52, 57, 72, 78, 96, 122, 133, 134, 137, 154, 158, 181
community, xxi, xxii, 2, 4, 5, 6, 9, 10, 12, 13, 22, 42, 43, 44, 45, 47, 48, 52, 57, 58, 59, 69, 70, 71, 72, 76, 78, 81, 88, 89, 90, 92, 93, 94, 98, 139, 146, 181, 187, 191, 207, 211, 213, 227, 232, 236, 248
community service, 4, 57, 58, 59, 236
Community-based Positive Youth Development, 196
community-based positive youth program, 22
Community-based Youth Enhancement Program, 171
comparative method, 17
compassion, 16, 17
compassionate, 188
compensation, 157
competencies, 22, 98, 99, 100, 109, 113, 114, 122, 123, 124, 138, 147, 148, 152, 158, 162, 163, 164, 169, 204

conceptualization, 113, 196, 200, 202, 204, 206
concerned, 3, 152, 171, 188
confidentiality, 53, 77
conflict resolution, 59, 87, 91, 155
congruence, 123
conscientiousness, 129
consciousness, 247
consent, 77, 101, 127, 128, 150, 151, 174, 199, 215
construction, 120, 143
content analysis, 195, 201, 211, 215, 227
convenience sample, 199
cooperation, 23, 55, 59, 80, 81, 82, 104, 122, 132, 134, 135, 137, 146, 149, 158, 161, 180, 204, 212, 216, 219, 221, 223
cooperative learning, 63, 66
cope, 11, 18, 50, 182, 183, 212
coping, 12, 31, 182, 183, 184
coping strategies, 183, 184
correlation coefficient, 175, 178
counseling, 4, 113, 119, 124, 142, 143, 148, 149, 152, 162, 163, 167, 211, 232
creativity, 64, 74, 80, 83, 129, 139, 207, 216, 223
criticism, 113, 151, 186, 205
culture, 60, 63, 82, 167, 204, 246
curriculum, 27, 44, 66, 92, 106, 112, 124, 148, 190, 191, 192, 196, 226

D

data analysis, 119, 143, 166, 175, 214, 217, 225, 227, 246
data collection, 33, 127, 139, 170, 173, 175, 176, 189, 214, 218
debriefing, 17, 60, 63, 72, 75, 87, 91, 206, 212, 224
decision-making process, 187
delinquency, 146, 167
delinquent behavior, 3

dementia, 31, 42, 43
demographic characteristics, 166
demographic data, 173, 199
Denmark, 232, 242
depression, 44, 146, 167, 223, 227
depressive symptoms, 32, 223, 227
depth, 5, 23, 24, 53, 101, 164, 220, 221, 224, 225
development, xxi, xxiii, 2, 5, 10, 11, 12, 13, 16, 17, 22, 23, 25, 26, 30, 31, 32, 40, 43, 44, 48, 50, 51, 52, 56, 58, 63, 65, 66, 70, 72, 73, 74, 75, 81, 82, 85, 93, 94, 95, 96, 98, 99, 100, 102, 108, 109, 113, 114, 115, 116, 118, 119, 121, 122, 123, 124, 125, 128, 137, 138, 139, 140, 141, 142, 143, 148, 153, 162, 163, 165, 167, 168, 170, 171, 174, 179, 180, 182, 185, 186, 187, 188, 190, 191, 192, 193, 196, 200, 206, 207, 210, 211, 212, 215, 221, 223, 224, 232, 236, 240, 242, 245, 249
developmental change, 183
developmental process, 224
developmental resources, 204
developmental risks, 187
deviant affiliation theory, 162
disability, 181, 232, 239, 240, 242
disadvantaged students, 66, 96
distribution, 87, 201, 203, 217
diversity, 139, 156
division of labor, 80, 82
DOI, 6, 26, 27, 42, 120, 142, 168, 190, 191, 192, 207, 208, 226, 227
dream, 106, 112, 129, 130, 131
drug abuse, 49
drug addiction, 49
drugs, 49

E

eating disorders, 246, 249
economic disadvantage, 150
economic status, 204
educational, 67, 86, 98, 99, 104, 138, 150, 197, 204, 205, 213
educational settings, 213
educators, 41, 115, 140, 147
effectiveness, 5, 11, 12, 33, 35, 38, 47, 53, 55, 57, 63, 66, 76, 79, 81, 83, 84, 86, 89, 91, 92, 93, 94, 96, 118, 122, 128, 138, 141, 146, 148, 149, 151, 152, 161, 163, 165, 171, 172, 179, 189, 195, 198, 204, 209, 210, 211, 213, 219, 223
egocentrism, 11, 25
elderly, 18, 19, 21, 31, 32, 42, 43, 53, 57, 59, 72, 73, 146, 148, 149, 154, 155, 156, 157, 158, 159, 161, 180, 181, 185, 188, 198, 211, 232
elementary school, 32, 44, 67, 96
emotion, 40, 50, 52, 183
emotion regulation, 50, 52
emotional, 49, 51, 52, 61, 89, 123, 152, 154, 157, 161, 170, 176, 182, 183, 184, 187, 192, 196, 210, 211, 213, 216, 222, 224, 227, 228
emotional attachment, 187
emotional competence, 52, 123, 152, 161, 170, 176, 182, 184, 192, 210
emotional experience, 183
emotional intelligence, 213, 227
emotional management, 154, 157, 182, 211, 216, 222
emotional problems, 61, 89, 157
emotional state, 183
empathy, 132, 156, 158, 180, 183, 222
empirical studies, 41, 162
empowerment, 23, 45, 147
encouragement, 31, 74, 75, 139, 164, 188, 219
English, 57, 197, 199
environment, 20, 22, 31, 32, 40, 44, 45, 74, 92, 114, 123, 131, 147, 163, 184
environmental awareness, 44
environments, 43, 45

ethical implications, 250
ethical standards, 180, 181
ethics, 73, 95, 248
etiquette, 151
everyday life, 21, 40, 53
evidence, 3, 10, 24, 26, 33, 43, 81, 93, 122, 124, 146, 162, 163, 248
evidence-based program, 3
examinations, 70, 103
exercise, 27, 43, 80, 125, 126, 131, 139, 148
Experiential learning, 66, 107, 113, 119, 198, 206, 207
experiential learning cycle, 200
experiential learning theory, 196, 198, 205
experimental design, 67, 226
exposure, 32, 50, 58, 148, 149, 154, 203
external environment, 129
externalizing behavior, 3, 146
extracurricular activities, 189
extrinsic rewards, 212

F

families, 12, 50, 192, 204
family life, 95
family members, 146, 155, 159, 161, 163, 187, 188
family socialization theory, 162
family support, 232
fear, 10, 205, 212
feelings, 23, 51, 62, 75, 79, 127, 132, 139, 149, 154, 164, 182, 205, 212
fidelity, 70
filial obedience, 188
filial piety, 188
flexibility, 150, 183, 184
Focus group, 5, 6, 10, 13, 15, 16, 18, 19, 23, 24, 30, 47, 53, 54, 55, 56, 58, 62, 70, 77, 81, 85, 86, 87, 88, 89, 90, 91, 98, 100, 101, 114, 119, 122, 127, 139, 140, 142, 143, 145, 149, 150, 151, 152, 158, 161, 162, 163, 165, 166, 167, 169, 173, 174, 175, 176, 188, 195, 198, 199, 200, 201, 205, 214
focus group interview, 5, 10, 13, 15, 16, 18, 19, 23, 30, 47, 53, 54, 55, 56, 58, 62, 70, 77, 81, 85, 86, 88, 89, 90, 91, 98, 101, 114, 127, 139, 149, 151, 161, 163, 170, 173, 174, 175, 176, 189, 195, 198, 199, 200, 201, 214
food, 81, 82, 156, 159
force, 20, 74, 86, 220
foul language, 155, 158
foundations, 192
fractures, 250
frequency distribution, 218
friendship, 56, 188
funding, 71, 171, 210
fundraising, 18

G

generalizability, 188
Germany, 207, 242
gerontology, 240
globalization, 250
goal setting, 50, 99, 103
goal-directed behavior, 62
goal-setting, 52
greater psychosocial needs, 1, 2, 4, 5, 6, 12, 30, 33, 41, 44, 50, 72, 73, 120, 124, 142, 146, 147, 148, 163, 168, 171, 172, 190, 191, 196, 198, 207, 213
greed, 104
green-based programs, 41
group activities, 73, 224
group work, 63, 162, 232
grouping, 152, 195, 197, 202, 203, 204, 207, 208
growth, 30, 31, 32, 38, 62, 64, 72, 74, 81, 83, 122, 134, 162, 210, 212, 223
guidance, 99, 114, 119, 138, 139, 142

H

happiness, 32, 50, 130
head and neck cancer, 250
healing, 31, 43, 45, 248
health, 6, 30, 39, 42, 43, 44, 45, 139, 142, 180, 190, 232, 239, 242, 245, 246, 247, 248, 249
health care, 42, 247
health education, 142
health effects, 246
high school, 33, 70, 167
higher education, 192, 250
holistic, 4, 12, 25, 32, 41, 64, 70, 98, 113, 114, 122, 140, 146, 147, 166, 170, 196, 208, 210, 247, 248, 249
holistic development, 4, 32, 122, 146, 170, 210
holistic medicine, 247
holistic youth development, 113, 196
holistic youth programs, 41
Hong Kong, xv, xxii, 1, 2, 4, 6, 9, 10, 11, 12, 14, 24, 25, 26, 29, 31, 42, 45, 47, 48, 51, 52, 64, 69, 70, 71, 76, 82, 88, 93, 95, 96, 97, 98, 99, 100, 105, 112, 114, 115, 119, 121, 122, 124, 138, 139, 140, 143, 145, 146, 148, 149, 150, 161, 163, 164, 166, 167, 169, 170, 188, 190, 191, 192, 195, 196, 197, 198, 206, 207, 208, 209, 210, 225, 226, 227, 231, 232, 235, 236, 242, 247
horticultural therapy, xxi, 29, 30, 32, 40, 41, 42, 43, 44
hospitality, 105, 110
hotel, 105, 110, 111, 126
human, xxiii, 26, 30, 42, 45, 95, 123, 166, 179, 212, 232, 235, 240, 242, 245, 249
human capital, 212
human development, xxiii, 26, 123, 232, 240, 242, 245, 249
humbleness, 188

hypothesis, 205, 225

I

ideal, 3, 32, 70, 95
identification, 109, 226
identity, 23, 52, 70, 72, 75, 78, 83, 102, 123, 131, 138, 143, 152, 154, 171, 179, 184, 210
imagination, 80
immigrants, 150
immunodeficiency, 248
improvements, 23, 58, 157, 176, 179, 180, 187
impulsive, 132
inadequate social skills, 172
independence, 12, 98, 138, 192
indigenous knowledge, 236
individual differences, 41
individual students, 197
individuals, 10, 11, 30, 32, 51, 62, 63, 74, 98, 99, 113, 139, 187, 212
inequality, 208, 225
inferiority, 153, 154
informed consent, 16, 53, 199
Informed verbal consents, 199
integration, 14, 72, 123, 138, 168, 245
intelligence, 74, 213, 227
intention, 200, 204, 205
interaction, 24, 30, 31, 36, 37, 40, 41, 53, 63, 113, 147, 184, 186, 206
interdependence, 63
interim evaluation, 171, 210
inter-judgmental agreement, 196, 201
internalizing, 3, 146
interpersonal attitude, 50
interpersonal communication, 80, 82, 154
interpersonal competence, 122, 134, 137
interpersonal conflicts, 179, 180
interpersonal relationship, 10, 39, 40, 49, 83, 150, 179, 180, 183, 223

interpersonal relationships, 39, 40, 49, 150, 183, 223
interpersonal skills, 14, 41, 50, 56, 58, 63, 81, 219
Inter-rater reliability, 170, 175
intervention, 4, 12, 27, 31, 32, 40, 45, 52, 65, 87, 92, 94, 99, 100, 113, 116, 124, 139, 147, 148, 163, 164, 209, 223
intervention strategies, 116, 124, 148
intimacy, 138
intrapersonal development, 90, 109, 124, 137
intrinsic, 62, 185, 212
intrinsic motivation, 62
intrinsic value, 62
Israel, xxiii, 2, 232, 239, 240, 242, 243, 250
issues, 16, 19, 25, 43, 70, 71, 82, 146, 151, 166

K

knowledge, 2, 27, 37, 44, 49, 51, 72, 91, 122, 125, 153, 157, 170, 185, 187, 189, 204, 236
knowledge transfer, 204

L

lack of control, 64
leadership, 12, 14, 73, 74, 75, 76, 78, 81, 90, 91, 95, 131, 213, 216, 223, 227
leadership development, 74, 95
learning disabilities, 167
learning environment, 10, 41
learning outcomes, xxii, 63, 66, 195, 196, 198, 206
learning process, 51, 162, 196, 201
life and career development, xxii, 98, 99, 100, 101, 102, 112, 113, 114, 115, 119, 122, 123, 124, 125, 127, 128, 137, 138, 139

Life career development, 119, 123, 142
life course, 100, 125
life cycle, 95, 187, 192
life experiences, 51, 172
life satisfaction, 11, 167
life tasks, 185
Likert scale, 33, 36, 37, 38
living environment, 31
loneliness, 167
longitudinal research, 173, 205, 210
longitudinal study, 45, 167, 169, 191, 207, 210, 214, 215, 223
love, 188
low-achieving students, xxii, 145, 148, 149, 162, 163, 164, 167

M

majority, 35, 40, 59, 82, 124, 158, 171, 212
management, 23, 70, 88, 90, 99, 105, 110, 130, 154, 157, 182, 211, 213, 216, 222, 223, 247, 249
manpower, 88, 89, 92, 114, 139, 164, 189
materialism, 25
materials, 71, 80, 82, 86, 91, 108, 111, 131, 215
Mathematics, 197
mediating role, 172
medical, 232, 247
medicine, 147, 242, 245, 248
medium of instruction, 197, 199
mental disorder, 2, 3, 247
mental health, 26, 43, 45, 99
mentor program, 43
meta-analysis, 208
methodology, 5, 24, 100, 122, 127, 145, 152, 163
migration, 236, 247
Millennials, 98, 118
models, 26, 99, 111, 114, 200
mood disorder, 247

moral behavior, 191
moral competence, 52, 56, 71, 72, 123, 152, 161, 170, 210
moral development, 189
moral reasoning, 224, 228
motivation, 21, 56, 58, 61, 62, 66, 92, 114, 124, 126, 139, 147, 150, 158, 167, 187, 207
MSW, 9, 29, 169, 195, 208, 232
multicultural education, 67
multidimensional, 183
mutual help, 63, 180
mutual learning, 204
mutual respect, 85, 87, 110, 111
mycotoxins, 246

N

narratives, 17, 98, 104, 105, 106, 107, 108, 109, 110, 111, 112
needy, 52, 147, 181, 186, 211
negative emotions, 136, 182, 183
neglect, 155, 159, 246
neutral, 128, 152
New South Wales, 43
next generation, 118, 242
normal development, 147
normative behavior, 186, 187
null hypothesis, 217, 227
nursing, 31, 42, 43
nursing home, 31, 42, 43
nurturance, 73

O

obedience, 188
opportunities, 12, 14, 21, 53, 56, 64, 81, 99, 100, 114, 124, 129, 138, 153, 155, 171, 181, 185
optimism, 12, 23, 183, 192
optimistic, 18, 22, 129, 131, 184, 212

organize, 59, 73
ornamental plants, 45

P

pain, v, viii, xiii, xvi, xvii, 192, 246
parental consent, 174, 214
parental control, 232
parents, 10, 11, 13, 15, 19, 22, 24, 33, 54, 70, 75, 76, 95, 98, 101, 106, 127, 150, 158, 161, 162, 172, 187, 188, 192, 199, 213
participants, 4, 5, 6, 10, 12, 13, 15, 16, 18, 19, 22, 23, 24, 26, 30, 31, 33, 34, 36, 37, 39, 40, 41, 42, 43, 47, 48, 49, 50, 52, 54, 55, 57, 59, 62, 63, 64, 65, 66, 70, 72, 73, 74, 75, 76, 77, 78, 79, 80, 81, 82, 83, 85, 87, 89, 90, 92, 93, 94, 95, 98, 100, 101, 102, 103, 115, 116, 117, 124, 127, 128, 139, 140, 149, 150, 151, 152, 158, 163, 164, 169, 171, 172, 173, 174, 176, 179, 180, 181, 182, 183, 184, 185, 187, 188, 190, 196, 198, 199, 200, 201, 202, 204, 205, 206, 209, 211, 212, 213, 214, 215, 217, 218, 219, 220, 221, 222, 223, 224, 225, 226
pathology-oriented clinical intervention, 147
pathways, 27, 99
peer conflict, 146
peer culture, 204
peer group, 61
peer relationship, 12, 50, 138, 216, 222, 223, 224
peers, 16, 17, 23, 49, 75, 133, 146, 156, 161, 167, 187, 188
perceptions, 13, 15, 22, 23, 35, 40, 51, 55, 79, 95, 149, 163, 174, 183, 191, 215
perceptions of control, 183
perseverance, 184, 185
personal development, 16, 81, 99, 221

personal life, 122
personal styles, 123
personality, 75, 99, 208
physical activity, 22, 25, 27
physical health, 32
physiological arousal, 40
planning for action, 196, 198, 200, 202, 205
plants, 30, 34, 35, 40, 44, 45
policy, 43, 90, 91, 95, 208, 242
population, 32, 44, 53
positive attitudes, 109
positive behaviors, 61
positive characters, 186, 187
positive feedback, 61, 64, 75, 85, 171
positive relationship, 19, 110
positive youth development, xxi, xxii, 4, 6, 9, 10, 11, 12, 13, 17, 22, 23, 25, 26, 27, 29, 44, 47, 50, 52, 71, 72, 76, 90, 93, 95, 96, 98, 99, 100, 101, 102, 109, 112, 114, 115, 116, 119, 122, 123, 124, 127, 128, 137, 138, 139, 140, 142, 145, 146, 148, 152, 162, 163, 164, 167, 168, 169, 170, 174, 190, 191, 192, 195, 199, 207, 208, 209, 210, 211, 225, 226, 227, 232, 246
positive youth development program, xxi, xxii, 4, 6, 9, 10, 12, 13, 23, 25, 26, 27, 44, 47, 90, 93, 95, 96, 122, 124, 142, 145, 146, 148, 162, 163, 164, 167, 168, 169, 190, 191, 195, 207, 208, 209, 226, 227
potential benefits, 41
poverty, 88, 168, 232
predictive validity, 227
preparation, xx, 6, 12, 24, 64, 79, 88, 91, 92, 99, 108, 109, 115, 138, 140, 164, 190, 206, 225
prevention, 2, 3, 4, 6, 22, 167, 171, 172, 190, 198, 208, 210, 232, 247
primary school, 179, 186, 197, 205
principles, 17, 42, 109, 110, 130, 248
problem behavior, 2, 3, 146, 147, 162, 166, 167

problem behavior theory, 162
problem solving, 10, 35, 49, 75
problem-focused coping, 12
problem-solving, 14, 57, 80, 81, 100, 104, 105, 125, 126, 153, 157, 211, 216, 222, 223, 224
process evaluation, 65, 171
professionals, 75, 198, 235, 240, 242
program design, 33, 59, 62, 63, 65, 70, 86, 90, 91, 94, 98, 101, 102, 103, 124, 139, 148, 162, 170, 196, 206
program implementer(s), 5, 6, 10, 13, 15, 16, 22, 24, 30, 35, 37, 48, 53, 54, 55, 56, 57, 63, 66, 76, 77, 78, 81, 82, 83, 84, 85, 86, 87, 88, 89, 90, 91, 92, 95, 98, 100, 101, 171, 189, 191, 206, 207, 226
program outcomes, 3, 15
program participants, 4, 5, 6, 10, 13, 15, 18, 22, 23, 24, 47, 52, 66, 70, 85, 95, 171, 174, 189, 200, 204, 205, 209, 226
program staff, 76, 94
project, xxii, 2, 4, 5, 12, 44, 48, 64, 69, 71, 78, 88, 122, 124, 127, 128, 129, 139, 152, 170, 196, 204, 226, 237
Project P.A.T.H.S., 4, 5, 6, 12, 24, 42, 48, 50, 52, 55, 61, 64, 66, 70, 71, 75, 76, 81, 91, 93, 94, 95, 100, 101, 102, 109, 115, 116, 117, 119, 122, 124, 127, 128, 137, 140, 143, 146, 148, 149, 150, 160, 161, 164, 167, 170, 172, 190, 191, 195, 196, 197, 198, 199, 205, 206, 207, 208, 210, 211, 225, 226
propagation, 34
prosocial behavior, 180, 212
prosocial involvement, 12, 123, 152, 163, 171, 176, 180, 181, 210
prosocial norms, 72, 123, 152, 162, 170, 176, 180, 210
prosocial orientation, 186
protection, 174, 199, 214
protective factors, 3, 183, 187, 223, 227
psychiatric illness, 45

psychiatry, 247, 249
psychological well-being, 30, 32, 40, 41, 43
psychology, 26, 27, 67, 142, 143, 147, 166, 191, 235, 246
psychometric properties, 5, 25
psychopharmacology, 247
psychosocial, xxi, 3, 4, 22, 41, 71, 75, 98, 102, 108, 109, 113, 116, 124, 137, 138, 140, 148, 149, 152, 163, 167, 172, 196, 213, 226
psychosocial development, 98, 102, 108, 109, 116, 138, 140, 167
psychosocial needs, xxi, 4, 41, 71, 149, 163, 172, 213, 226
psycho-social-moral development, 189
psychotherapy, 30
public administration, 207
public health, 232, 239, 240, 242, 245, 246, 248, 249
public housing, 157
public service, 240

Q

Qualitative, 5, 10, 12, 13, 23, 26, 27, 30, 32, 35, 41, 43, 53, 54, 64, 66, 70, 95, 98, 102, 114, 119, 122, 127, 128, 139, 142, 143, 145, 149, 151, 152, 162, 163, 166, 168, 171, 172, 173, 175, 191, 193, 196, 205, 209, 210, 211, 215, 226, 227
qualitative data, 10, 23, 35, 54, 98, 114, 139, 149, 163, 209, 227
qualitative evaluation, 33, 43, 114, 122, 145, 163, 210
qualitative outcome evaluation, 196
qualitative research, 5, 13, 26, 119, 127, 143, 166, 171, 172, 175, 205
quality of life, 32, 42, 44, 196, 204, 232, 246, 248, 249, 250

R

randomized controlled trial, 171
rapport, 205
real-life experiences, 172
reasoning, 70, 224
recall, 189, 203, 209, 215
reciprocity, 180
recognition, 21, 52, 63, 78, 123, 147, 152, 170, 171, 210
recognition for positive behavior, 152, 171, 210
recovery, 31, 45, 249
recruiting, 65, 94, 107
reflective observation, 113, 196, 200, 202, 203, 205
regulations, 147, 186
rehabilitation, 30, 31, 45, 232, 239
rejection, 205, 219
reliability, 96, 170, 175, 178, 201, 217
replication, 44, 142, 167, 168, 190
representativeness, 64
resilience, 52, 56, 75, 78, 80, 81, 99, 100, 104, 122, 123, 125, 137, 138, 147, 149, 152, 153, 157, 162, 163, 167, 170, 176, 183, 184, 192, 193, 210, 216, 218, 219, 221, 223, 224, 227, 232
resources, 3, 87, 89, 109, 146, 154, 183, 204, 205
response, 24, 33, 45, 50, 87, 176, 205, 221
responsibility, xx, 16, 17, 22, 44, 87, 180, 187, 212, 236
responsible, 72, 77, 82, 88, 89, 92, 94, 98, 142, 149, 179, 182, 232, 236
risk, 2, 3, 4, 32, 43, 168, 192, 211, 226, 227, 248
risk factors, 3
romantic partners, 187
rules, 87, 103, 151
rural areas, 149

S

school, 4, 10, 12, 13, 14, 15, 20, 21, 22, 23, 24, 32, 33, 34, 40, 41, 42, 44, 48, 50, 52, 53, 54, 58, 60, 61, 64, 65, 66, 71, 72, 73, 76, 78, 79, 80, 81, 82, 85, 86, 88, 89, 91, 92, 94, 96, 98, 99, 101, 108, 109, 111, 114, 115, 118, 119, 124, 127, 129, 133, 139, 141, 146, 147, 148, 149, 150, 151, 156, 161, 163, 165, 166, 167, 170, 171, 172, 173, 174, 175, 179, 183, 186, 187, 188, 191, 192, 193, 195, 196, 197, 198, 199, 201, 204, 205, 207, 208, 210, 213, 214, 225, 226, 232, 242
school activities, 14, 22
school adjustment, 167, 172, 213
school climate, 66, 166
school social work, 4, 24, 42, 50, 85, 101, 149, 151, 171, 173, 174, 188, 195, 198, 199, 204, 205, 214
school social workers, 4, 24, 42, 50, 85, 101, 149, 151, 174, 188, 195, 198, 199, 205, 214
schoolmates, 59, 86, 156, 187
school-to-work-to-life (STWL) intervention model, 99
science, 6, 190, 192, 210, 217, 235, 240, 248
secondary prevention program, 3, 4, 171, 172, 198
secondary school students, 4, 12, 13, 30, 32, 33, 40, 52, 71, 76, 85, 100, 124, 146, 148, 169, 207
secondary schools, 48, 52, 71, 72, 114, 119, 146, 150, 197
secondary students, 10, 195
secondary teachers, 207
self-actualization, 62
self-assessment, 51
self-awareness, 23, 49, 50, 213
self-concept, 75, 123, 212
self-confidence, 16, 17, 23, 49, 105, 122, 131, 134, 137, 150, 154, 162, 163, 184, 216, 218, 223
self-determination, 52, 103, 123, 143, 152, 170, 210, 216, 218, 220, 221, 224
self-discipline, 23, 210, 216, 218, 223
self-doubt, 138
self-efficacy, 49, 50, 52, 72, 78, 123, 128, 138, 152, 170, 172, 176, 183, 184, 185, 210, 213
self-esteem, 11, 32, 44, 50, 51, 58, 60, 61, 63, 66, 72, 76, 167, 172, 205, 213
self-harm behavior, 182, 183
self-identity, 98, 102, 109, 138, 147, 179, 180, 216, 223
self-image, 51, 60, 63
self-improvement, 60
self-perceptions, 23, 51
self-reflection, 63
self-regulation, 204, 207
self-reports, 55
self-understanding, 23, 32, 53, 99, 102, 113, 122, 123, 125, 132, 138, 216, 223
self-worth, 51
semi-structured interviews, 16, 209
service organization, 232
services, xx, 4, 26, 31, 56, 71, 72, 124, 148, 172, 173, 179, 185, 188, 211, 212, 213, 214, 221, 224, 232, 236
sharing, 39, 100, 103, 105, 106, 107, 108, 114, 124, 128, 130, 134, 139, 161, 170, 180, 183
shelter, 44
showing, 41, 53, 61, 124, 151, 162, 179, 222
siblings, 183, 187
simulation, 103, 113, 131, 139
simulation games, 103, 113
skills, 10, 11, 12, 14, 18, 19, 20, 23, 27, 32, 34, 35, 37, 39, 41, 44, 48, 49, 50, 52, 53, 56, 57, 58, 59, 60, 61, 62, 63, 64, 70, 72, 73, 74, 76, 78, 80, 81, 82, 83, 86, 90, 91,

96, 100, 116, 122, 125, 126, 130, 133, 134, 137, 153, 154, 158, 169, 181, 182, 185, 186, 187, 189, 193, 204, 205, 206, 208, 213, 216, 218, 219, 221, 222, 223, 224
skills training, 72, 73, 76, 208
social activities, 184
social behavior, 27
social benefits, 41
social change, 236
social circle, 49, 135
social competence, 41, 52, 123, 152, 170, 176, 179, 184, 187, 210
social context, 23
social desirability, 93
social development, 162, 167, 192, 193
social development model, 162, 167
social environment, 23
social exchange, 12
social group, 77
social impairment, 32
social justice, 208, 236
social knowledge, 186, 187
social network, 61, 212
social norms, 186
social policy, 235
social programs, 25, 166
social reality, 11
social relations, 22, 187
social relationships, 22, 187
social responsibility, 22
social services, 215
social skills, 18, 19, 23, 32, 49, 50, 61, 172, 186, 187, 213, 219, 221
social status, 11
social welfare, 173, 214, 231
social workers, 4, 13, 15, 21, 24, 42, 48, 50, 52, 53, 55, 58, 59, 60, 61, 62, 63, 64, 65, 70, 72, 73, 76, 77, 85, 88, 89, 90, 91, 92, 94, 101, 108, 115, 139, 140, 146, 147, 149, 151, 170, 172, 174, 188, 192, 195, 198, 199, 205, 213, 214, 224

socialization, 162
society, 11, 16, 17, 75, 95, 98, 100, 103, 104, 108, 112, 125, 138, 156, 163, 180, 236, 240
special education, 86
specific knowledge, 91
spirituality, 16, 17, 52, 123, 128, 152, 170, 189, 210
staff members, 91
stakeholders, 10, 16, 24, 54
standard of living, 161
statistics, 25, 34, 35, 202
strain theory, 162
strategy use, 208
Strengths-based orientation, 109
strengths-based perspective, 109, 147, 163
stress, 4, 31, 32, 40, 43, 44, 70, 74, 95, 183, 197
stress management, 4, 74
structure, 11, 25
structured after-school activities, 22
student achievement, 66, 207, 208
styles, 92, 110
subjective experience, 122, 139, 145, 150, 164
subjective outcome evaluation, 5, 6, 33, 45, 48, 54, 171, 190, 206
substance abuse, 2, 3, 12
substance use, 167, 208, 249
suicidal behavior, 3
suicidal ideation, 2, 3
suicide, 10, 25, 247
summer program, 60
Sun, 4, 6, 25, 26, 44, 66, 90, 92, 95, 96, 119, 142, 166, 167, 168, 190, 191, 208, 226, 247, 249
symptoms, viii, 32, 166, 248, 249

T

teachers, 4, 10, 13, 15, 16, 17, 19, 21, 48, 58, 61, 62, 63, 64, 70, 72, 73, 75, 76, 85, 87, 88, 89, 90, 91, 92, 96, 99, 101, 111, 114, 139, 146, 147, 149, 151, 156, 161, 162, 172, 187, 197, 207, 213
teacher-student relationship, 114, 166
team members, 219, 220
techniques, 26, 34, 48, 56, 60, 62, 63, 70, 72, 86, 87, 90, 91, 116, 139, 148
textbook, 197, 247
Thematic analysis, 170, 175
theme analysis pattern coding, 152
theory of change, 189
therapeutic benefits, 32
therapeutic change, 211
therapeutic community, 26
therapeutic effect, 31
therapist, 34, 40
therapy, xxi, 26, 29, 30, 31, 32, 40, 41, 42, 43, 44, 45, 72, 73, 246
therapy methods, 42
thoughts, 23, 75, 79, 82, 181, 182, 205, 212, 223
Tier 1, 4, 12, 50, 52, 55, 65, 71, 73, 76, 77, 79, 86, 87, 88, 89, 91, 92, 94, 124, 148, 171, 172, 190, 196, 213
Tier 1 program, 12, 55, 171, 172, 190
Tier 2 program, 5, 12, 13, 14, 21, 50, 52, 55, 77, 78, 80, 81, 82, 89, 116, 117, 148, 153, 160, 171, 172, 173, 179, 196, 198, 200, 205
training, 14, 25, 49, 53, 60, 63, 72, 73, 74, 75, 76, 77, 78, 81, 91, 96, 100, 103, 104, 106, 113, 116, 119, 124, 125, 132, 139, 166, 171, 174, 179, 183, 188, 196, 198, 199, 200, 203, 215, 220, 223, 232, 240
transcripts, 102, 128, 152
transition to adulthood, 2, 3, 138
treatment, 2, 3, 31, 247
trial, 171, 190
triangulation, 176, 189
trustworthiness, 17
tuberculosis, 248

U

underlying mechanisms, 166
United Kingdom, 236, 242
United States (USA), 1, 26, 27, 30, 74, 95, 97, 142, 167, 190, 226, 232, 236, 242

V

validation, 119, 142, 167, 192
validity, 33, 34, 188, 227
variables, 34, 201
verbatim, 17, 101, 102, 128, 151, 152, 176, 201
Vice President, 1, 9, 29, 231
violence, 3, 155, 162, 208, 227
visually impaired, 180, 181
vocational development, 123, 138
volunteer services, 148, 221, 224
volunteer training and service, 171, 179, 196, 203
volunteerism, 180

W

walking, 156, 159, 220
weakness, 147, 186
wealth, 130
welfare, 232, 239
well-being, 2, 3, 212, 233
whole-person development, 21, 99, 138
withdrawal, 146, 153
work environment, 103, 142

workers, 2, 3, 4, 32, 53, 54, 57, 59, 60, 63, 65, 70, 72, 77, 80, 81, 83, 84, 88, 89, 91, 92, 93, 101, 149, 151, 199
workload, 88, 92
written informed consents, 199

Y

young adults, 227
young people, xxi, 1, 3, 5, 10, 20, 50, 73, 210, 211
youth prevention programs, 4